THE
BLACK MAN'S
GUIDE TO
GOOD HEALTH

THE
BLACK MAN'S
GUIDE TO
GOOD HEALTH

ESSENTIAL ADVICE
FOR THE SPECIAL CONCERNS
OF AFRICAN-AMERICAN MEN

James W. Reed, M.D., F.A.C.P.,
Neil B. Shulman, M.D.,
and Charlene Shucker

A PERIGEE BOOK

A Perigee Book
Published by The Berkley Publishing Group
200 Madison Avenue
New York, NY 10016

Book design by Stanley S. Drate/Folio Graphics Co. Inc.

Cover design by Judith Murello

First edition: October 1994

Published simultaneously in Canada.

*This book is not intended as a substitute for the medical advice
of physicians. The reader should regularly consult a physician
about matters relating to his or her health and particularly
regarding any symptom that may require diagnosis or medical
attention.*

Library of Congress Cataloging-in-Publication Data

Reed, James W.
    The black man's guide to good health : essential advice for the
special concerns of African-American men / by James W. Reed, M.D.,
Neil B. Shulman, M.D., and Charlene Shucker. — 1st Perigee ed.
        p.   cm.
    ISBN 0-399-52138-0
    1. Afro-American men—Health and hygiene.   2. Afro-American
men—Diseases.   I. Shulman, Neil.   II. Shucker, Charlene.
III. Title.
RA777.8.R44   1994
613′.04234′08996073—dc20   94-13443
                                                        CIP

PRINTED IN THE UNITED STATES OF AMERICA

10   9   8   7   6   5   4   3   2

Medical literacy is the missing link in quality health care. Health education is just as important as the three R's, for without health, it's difficult to read, write, or do arithmetic.

—NEIL SHULMAN

CONTENTS

A GUIDE TO
TABLES AND FIGURES

Chapter 8: Kidney Disease

Chapter 9: AIDS and Sexually Transmitted Diseases

ACKNOWLEDGMENTS

Our heartfelt thanks go to the physicians, nurses, researchers and other professionals who personally shared their knowledge with us: Michael Kell, Thomas Hestor, Keith Woods, Sharni Sheehy, Hugh Moore, Gurinderjit Sidhu, Bruce Herschatter, John Ambri, Charles Gilbert, Charles Francis, Barry Silverman, William Mitch, Mark Stephen Travis, Joe Havlik, James Delcher, Mark Rosenberg, James Hunter, Stephanie Fox, Cathy Schnell, Lane Harrison, Debra Mlambo, Ira Bragg, Stacy Pelisero, Mary Stewart, David Grant, Joyce Dittmer, Ms. Thomas, Trish Grindell, Katheryn Tauber, Ira Schwartz, Kathy Berkowitz, Deb Sanden, Mae Clayton, Julie Feltham, Polly Clary, Melanie McLeod, Cam Langston, Lynn Humphrey and Patti Moore.

We especially want to thank all the patients and families who educated us about their personal experiences, which helped us to develop the fictional case studies in this book. All names have been changed. We wish them many years of health and happiness. We also wish to thank those who gave us permission to use previously published figures to illustrate our text.

Although there are only three names on the cover of this book, the completed work could never have occurred without the consistent and diligent writing, editing and proofreading talents of Robin Voss and Laurie E. Smith. Thank you is not enough, but they are the only two words in the English language that come close to expressing our gratitude. In addition, Letitia Sweitzer and Lynn Aaron were invaluable members of the team, whose efforts went way beyond the call of duty.

Putting this book together was no easy task. All of the participants had other commitments, but were willing to sacrifice their time and talents and devote their energies to this project because we believed it to be so worthwhile. No one was more dedicated than the four women mentioned above. During the toughest times they provided inspiration, pep talks and humor. We hope that as the years come and go, you will always be a part of our lives as critics, confidantes and friends.

THE
BLACK MAN'S
GUIDE TO
GOOD HEALTH

1

An Overview

Black men in America live an average of seventy years, while white men live an average of seventy-three years. We have access to the same doctors, hospitals and health care as other racial groups, but we contract more diseases and die earlier than our white counterparts. As a group, we may see ourselves as very diverse. After all, our ancestors hailed from different origins, we live in different parts of the country and we each have different hopes, dreams and desires. Yet, for some reason, the color of our skin—especially for black *men*—means we are more likely to experience a greater amount of pain and suffering than our friends in other racial groups, particularly when it comes to health care.

Good health is a frame of mind. Unfortunately, we often think of health in negative terms. When we're healthy, we think, "It couldn't happen to me," or "My body is strong enough to take care of itself—it doesn't need any help." When we get sick, however, we change our tune and we're willing to do whatever it takes to get our health back. We allow doctors and nurses to stick us with needles, cut us, put tubes down our throats, into our stomachs or up our rectums. When we lose control of our bodies, we'll suddenly go to extremes to become "cured." Sometimes, the effort comes too late. By putting a little effort toward prevention now, we can save ourselves from endless suffering later.

In the grand scheme of things, life is a relatively short journey. Sometimes we get so busy trying to earn a living that we forget to take proper care of our health. Proper care of the body, however, can improve the quality of everyday living and give us more time to earn a living *and* to do those things we enjoy most.

Most men—not just black men—are hesitant to seek medical care on a regular basis. Unlike women, who often go to the doctor readily when a health problem arises, many men wait until they have a whole string of problems before seeking help. When our physical problems remain untreated, they often become worse, leading to more serious complications.

As men, we tend to believe that admitting we have health problems is the same as admitting weakness. Yet, in reality, seeing a doctor on a regular basis may be the strongest, smartest thing we do for ourselves. By making regular checkups a part of our lives, we may save ourselves and our loved ones from unnecessary suffering.

Naturally, it's much easier to talk about making changes than to actually take action. When we lead hectic lives, it can be difficult to find time to exercise or plan healthy meals. Living healthy can take extra time and energy—something few of us have. After reading this book, however, we hope you'll realize it will be time and effort well spent.

Knowledge is the cure

So how do we motivate ourselves? The first step is to become medically literate, to learn some medicine. Sometimes it seems as if doctors speak in a foreign language. Learning about medicine can seem complicated, at best. In reality, however, learning about the human body may be easier and more interesting than you realize. After all, when we learn about medicine, we are really learning about ourselves.

Have you ever wondered what your doctor sees when he or she looks into your eyes? What the different sounds of your heart are all about? Or how your brain is able to control all your body's functions? The answers to these mysteries are intriguing. It can be very interesting to learn how the human body works. Once you have accomplished this, you can then become empowered to take care of your own health.

When we learned about our rights as citizens of America during the civil rights movement, we became empowered to make changes. Now it's time for us to become empowered again. This time, we must make changes that have to do with one of the most important issues ever—saving our own lives. This book is a stepping stone toward overcoming the inequalities in our health system. As black men, we don't have to have the highest death rate or the greatest amount of suffering from disease. But we do.

"Why?" you may ask. The answer is far from simple. As you will see, some diseases, such as sickle cell anemia, are more common among blacks because of hereditary factors. Other diseases, like high blood pressure and heart disease, are more prevalent and fatal for black men because of our lifestyles, which include diets high in salt, fat and cholesterol. If we oversimplified the reasons for the inequalities you experience in health care, however, we would be doing you a great disservice.

For some of the diseases we'll discuss, there is no proven cause for these inequalities—we can only take an educated guess. For other diseases, the answer is a combination of many factors, including poor access to medical care, poverty, discrimination and a lack of research and awareness.

In each of the chapters that follow, we have addressed these issues more completely. However, we believe that more important than the question "Why?" is the question "What can we do about it?"

With recent advances in medical research, some diseases can now be prevented through diet, exercise, stress reduction, and early detection and treatment. Yet these things don't just happen. In order to reverse the statistics, we must each take control of our own health care. Instead of waiting for disease to strike, we need to prevent it before it has a chance. To do that, we must be informed. This book is a first step in that process.

We *can* reverse the statistics and become role models of healthy living for the rest of the world to follow.

How can this book help?

The Black Man's Guide to Good Health should serve as a catalyst in this effort. Ideally, you will read the book from start to finish, and learn about the challenges that are our highest priorities and the medical problems that cause us the most suffering. It's time to face the enemy, uncover its weakness and charge forward in conquest. This book should help you get behind enemy lines and learn about the internal workings of your body and how strokes, heart attacks and cancer weaken our bodies like villains. Why do certain diseases appear to unfairly ravage the body of a healthy black man? What makes your small blood vessels, which provide nourishment to your heart, clog? Why do normal healthy cells in your prostate gland or lung turn evil and spread cancer throughout your body? What makes the wall of an artery in your brain so weak it bursts?

Medical research has begun to unravel these mysteries. Studies now reveal that there are things we can do to prevent these internal mishaps. First, we can avoid the poisonous substances that destroy the inner workings of our bodies. Second, we can stretch our muscles and move our bodies, while enjoying sports that strengthen our healthy cells. Third, we can choose activities, friendships and work environments that keep our minds calm and peaceful, making it easier for us to maintain a positive state of health.

Even if we have inherited a predisposition to a certain disease through our genes, we can still take many actions to prevent or treat illness. Medical advances can now cure even hereditary illnesses. Dialysis machines can replace diseased kidneys. Heart specialists can open clogged blood vessels without surgical intervention. Chemicals, radiation and surgery are very often effective in destroying cancerous cells while maintaining healthy ones. Your doctor now has the tools to detect many medical disorders before they've progressed too far. The more you understand treatment options that are available, the better equipped you will be to choose the right specialist and make certain you are receiving the most advanced and effective remedy available.

The following chapters highlight preventive approaches to improving your health and reducing your risk of succumbing to the major killers of black men. Exercise, motivational techniques and good nutrition are just a few of the ways you can reduce your risk of disease. We've also included stories that focus on the real heroes, men who have discovered their illness at an early stage and taken action to control its progression, or cured themselves completely. We've listed additional references for more extensive reading, including names, addresses and phone numbers of nonprofit organizations that can provide you with the support, education and supplemental resources you may need.

If you read this book from cover to cover, you will gain the medical knowledge you need about how your body works and what can go wrong with it. You will learn about the staggering statistics that demonstrate how far black men's health status is from that of other groups in the population, and theories on why this difference exists. These theories span a wide spectrum of thought, from hereditary factors relating to slave trafficking across the Atlantic Ocean in the 18th and 19th centuries, to why darker skin correlates with higher blood pressure.

Read, learn and live a healthier life.

♦

2

Taking Control of Your Health

The first step in taking control of your health is living a healthy lifestyle. Everything you put into and do with your body has a direct impact on your health. It's important for us all to take good care of our bodies, not only when we're sick and trying to get better, but also when we're *healthy*. By making simple lifestyle changes, patients have found many ways to improve their health, from lowering high blood pressure to helping to prevent cancer.

This chapter discusses simple tips you can use to arm yourself against disease. When you eat right and exercise, you build your defenses against illness. This means you equip your body with the fuel it needs to heal itself of disease and prevent illness from taking its toll. Making change is never easy. When it comes to your health, however, changing your lifestyle may be a matter of life or death. By starting with these simple guidelines for good health, you will already be on your way to a healthier, happier life.

Eat a healthy diet

One theory of why black men are more susceptible to certain illnesses is diet. Traditional Southern food is often saltier and higher in fat than that of the North. While blacks are certainly from all areas of the U.S., many of our ancestors, at one time or another, lived in the South. Our families may have lived in the North or the West for years, but the traditional Southern diet may still have an influence on the way we eat today.

Salt contributes to high blood pressure, a disorder that can lead to fatal consequences like heart attacks, kidney failure or stroke. Fat clogs our arteries and may also contribute to heart disease, stroke, and complications of diabetes and high blood pressure.

Often, we get so busy, we have no time to make a home-cooked meal for ourselves or our families. Instead, we may stop at a fast food restaurant on the way home from work or pick up a frozen TV dinner at the supermarket. While these meals may be convenient, they are also often high in fat, calories, salt, sugar and cholesterol.

Instead of depending on foods already prepared for you, try following these simple guidelines to eating a healthy diet. You may find that eating right is easier and more delicious than you thought!

BUY MORE OFTEN . . .

Lean cuts of meat, poultry, fish

Skim or 1% milk

Low-fat cottage cheese, low-fat yogurt

Part-skim milk cheeses (like part-skim mozzarella)

Vegetable oils

Margarine

Plain fresh, frozen, or canned vegetables and fruit

Baking potatoes, rice, pasta

English muffins, bagels, loaf breads, tortillas, pita

Cold and hot cereals

BUY LESS OFTEN . . .

Fatty cuts of meat, breaded poultry or fish

Whole milk, cream

Cheese spreads and cheeses (like cheddar, American, Swiss)

Lard, butter, fat back, salt pork, shortening

Toppings (like butter, cheese sauces, gravy, sour cream)

Vegetables in cream or cheese sauces

French fries or hash browns

Doughnuts, Danish pastry

Desserts (like many cakes, cookies, and pies)

FIGURE 2A

How to shop for a healthier diet.
Reprinted from National Institute of Health: *Eat Right to Lower Your High Blood Cholesterol*, March 1992.

Eat foods low in saturated fat and "bad" cholesterol

When it comes to eating a healthy diet, it's important to learn to read food labels for content. The most important information to look for is fat and cholesterol content.

Always try to reduce the amount of fat you eat. There are two basic kinds of fats: saturated (bad) and unsaturated (good). Saturated fats clog your arteries and are unhealthy. If you *have* to eat fat, unsaturated is much better for your body.

Also check food labels to find out what kind of cholesterol they contain. Many people know their cholesterol level number (the target is under 200), but few know what it means. There are some good uses for cholesterol. It is a waxy, yellowish material found in your body's organs. Cholesterol is the foundation for all cell walls; it aids in digestion and produces hormones. However, as you probably know, cholesterol also has negative points—it can cause atherosclerosis (cholesterol buildup

TOTAL CHOLESTEROL	
<200 mg/dL	Desirable Blood Cholesterol
200–239 mg/dL	Borderline High Blood Cholesterol
≥240 mg/dL	High Blood Cholesterol

FIGURE 2B

Desirable range for total cholesterol.
Reprinted with permission from Merck: *Elevated Cholesterol—What It Means, What It Causes, What to Do About It.*

on the walls of your arteries), which can lead to cardio-vascular disease.

On the surface of your heart are three blood vessels that are the size of straws. If something the size of a pea (like cholesterol buildup) gets in one of these straws, it can close off the artery and cause a heart attack. "Bad" cholesterol (see below) can also break off from the surface

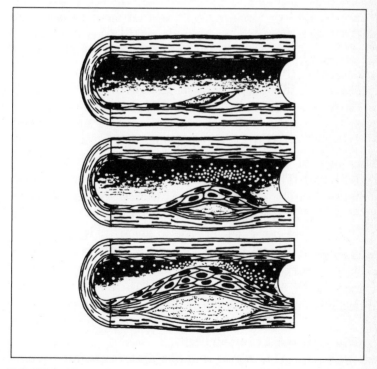

FIGURE 2C

How cholesterol forms on the wall of an artery.
Reprinted with permission from Merck: *Elevated Cholesterol—What It Means, What It Causes, What to Do About It.*

of your arteries and get into your bloodstream, blocking your smaller blood vessels entirely. Many studies have indicated that the higher your cholesterol level, the greater your risk of coronary heart disease and stroke.

Cholesterol is divided into two major groups: high-density lipoprotein and low-density lipoprotein. High-density lipoprotein (HDL) is considered the "good" type of cholesterol because it helps eliminate bad cholesterol from the circulatory system. The higher your HDL level, the lower your risk of a heart attack. Exercise may raise your HDL level. Smoking, on the other hand, lowers your HDL level. Low-density lipoprotein (LDL) is dangerous. This is the "bad" type of cholesterol. The higher your LDL level, the greater your risk of heart disease.

Maintaining a high ratio of "good" HDL to "bad" LDL is more important than lowering your overall cholesterol count. A ten-year study was conducted by the National Institutes of Health, which studied 3,806 men between the ages of 35 and 59, who had cholesterol levels above 265 mg/dl. This study confirmed that cholesterol in our diet is largely responsible for atherosclerosis. (We will discuss this type of heart disease further in Chapter Four.) "If we can get everyone to lower their cholesterol by 10 to 15 percent by cutting down on fat and cholesterol in their diet, heart attack deaths in this country will decrease by 30 percent," concluded Dr. Robert Levy, the cardiologist who helped coordinate the ten-year study.

When it comes to fat and cholesterol, here are some additional tips to remember:

◆ *Avoid eating butter and oils high in cholesterol and saturated fats.* Instead, choose a margarine with a liquid vegetable oil as the first ingredient. A tub of margarine contains more unsaturated (good) fat than a stick of margarine. Take advantage of the "light" margarines that are now available. Read the labels and choose one with as little fat and cholesterol as possible. Spend a couple of extra cents and save your body the cost of clogged arteries.

◆ *Use liquid vegetable oils whenever possible.* In recipes calling for one cup of solid shortening, substitute ¾ cup of liquid vegetable oil; replace ½ cup shortening with ⅓ cup vegetable oil. When cooking things on the stove or in a wok, use canola oil, which is made from the rape seed. This oil is lower in saturated fats than any other oil.

◆ *Use low-fat or non-fat dairy products.* While dairy products have been touted as healthy because they contain calcium, they can also have a high fat content. When eating dairy products, always try to choose low-fat options. Choose cheeses that have less than five grams of fat. Cheeses that are high in fat can add inches to your waistline and also clog your arteries. On the other hand, fat-free foods such as broccoli, tofu and leafy green vegetables can provide you with all the calcium your body needs. However, if you really enjoy dairy products, try low-fat options, such as skim milk or low-fat yogurt.

When cooking, substitute low-fat or non-fat dairy products for what is called for in a recipe. Low-fat or no-fat yogurt can be substituted for cream and mayonnaise.

◆ *Avoid eating egg yolks.* If you like eggs, check your supermarket for egg substitutes. These are very healthy because they contain egg whites with coloring, rather than egg yolks. (The yellow yolk in eggs is very high in saturated fats, while egg whites are high in protein and low in cholesterol.) You can use these mixes for baking or to make scrambled eggs or an omelet.

Another healthy alternative to eggs for breakfast is

Most recipes can be modified to reduce the amount of sugar, salt and/or fat called for in the ingredient list.

Here are some tips:

TO REDUCE SUGAR:

- Cut the amount of sugar called for by ½; reduce the amount of liquid by ¼.
- When fruit juice is called for, use apple juice and reduce the amount by ¼.
- Add a touch of vanilla flavoring or extract, or a dash of cinnamon, to a recipe calling for fruit to increase the sweet taste of the fruit.
- Heat up any low-sugar dessert prior to serving, when possible, to increase the sweet taste without adding sugar.

TO REDUCE SALT:

- Eliminate salt from all recipes (except those calling for yeast) and substitute herbs and spices instead. Here are some natural spice partners:

  Meat, fish, poultry: allspice, basil, sage, bay leaf, chives, dry mustard, lemon, garlic, onion and dill
  Vegetables: sesame seed, basil, oregano, allspice, ginger, tarragon, vinegar and lemon
  Fruit: cinnamon, cloves, vanilla, ginger, mint and nutmeg

TO REDUCE FAT:

- Select the leanest cuts of meat and use slower-cooking methods.
- Remove skin from poultry before serving.
- Allow dishes cooked in liquids to cool in refrigerator overnight, then skim off all visible fat.
- Use egg substitute or only egg whites in recipes that call for eggs. (Most but not all recipes can be modified this way.)

- Use liquid vegetable oil rather than solid shortening or butter.
- Use liquid margarine rather than solid margarine.
- Use skim milk rather than low-fat or whole milk.
- Use low-fat cheeses (farmer, ricotta) rather than high-fat cheeses (cheddar, American).
- Use protein-rich dried beans to substitute for meat in casseroles.

FIGURE 2D

Making recipes healthier.
Reprinted with permission of *Diabetes in the News*. Published by Miles, Inc., Diagnostics Division.

FOODS HIGH IN SATURATED FAT
Animal fats (such as butter, lard, beef and pork fat, fat back, salt pork, bacon and sausage grease)
Foods fried in animal fats
Gravy
Fatty meat (such as corned beef, regular ground beef, ribs, sausage, hot dogs, bacon, bologna, salami)
Whole milk, cream, ice cream
Most cheeses (such as cream cheese, cheddar, American, Swiss)
Cheese Danish
Many cakes, cookies, and pies

FOODS HIGH IN CHOLESTEROL
Egg yolks
Liver
Kidney

FIGURE 2E

Foods high in saturated fat and cholesterol.
Reprinted from National Institute of Health: *Eat Right to Lower Your High Blood Cholesterol*, March 1992.

fresh fruit. A fruit cup full of strawberries, grapes, bananas, melon and oranges can be a delicious and energizing way to start your day. If you can't give up eggs, limit your intake to no more than three per week. And choose egg whites over egg yolks.

Eat fresh vegetables

We may have hated this kind of food as children, but our mothers knew what they were talking about when they said, "Eat your vegetables." Like fruits, vegetables require little to no preparation. Most are as delicious raw as when they are cooked. Take a few carrots or celery sticks to work with you. They make a great snack! Vegetables are so easy to prepare. All you have to do is rinse (to remove pesticides), peel or cut to your liking and munch away! There are so many different kinds of vegetables—some that you may not even realize exist. If you think you hate vegetables, go to the supermarket and try something you've never eaten before.

Fresh vegetables are also delicious when mixed together in a salad. If you prefer cooked vegetables, steam them lightly over a pan of water or in the microwave. Make sure to cover them, to trap the steam and nutrients. Be careful not to overcook, though, because vegetables retain most of their flavor and nutrients only when they are cooked lightly. Avoid boiling or cooking vegetables with fat. Boiling and overcooking actually remove the good nutrients your body needs, and cooking with butter or oil can ruin the natural goodness of vegetables!

Also, always eat *fresh* vegetables whenever possible. Fresh vegetables are easy to prepare, delicious and healthy! Like fruits, they contain many vitamins that your immune system desperately needs to fight and prevent disease. When fresh vegetables are not available, use frozen because they are closest to fresh in terms of nutrient content. Canned vegetables may contain preservatives and tend to be high in sodium, although they can also be more affordable. If you prefer to buy canned vegetables, make sure you buy only those that are labeled *low in sodium.*

Eat more fresh fruit

There are very few people who don't like fruit. It's sweet, easy to eat and convenient. Best of all, fruit is one of the most healthy things you could ever eat! By eating a variety of fruits and vegetables, you can get many of the vitamins your body needs. Since there's *no* preparation involved, you can pick up a piece of fruit between appointments, on the way to work or as an evening snack.

Fruit is filled with natural carbohydrates and fiber. Your body desperately needs both of these to function properly and supply you with energy. Alone, fresh fruit is one of the healthiest things you can eat.

Eat whole grains

Whole-grain breads and pastas, and rice, beans and grains are the foundation of a good diet. When eating carbohydrates, such as pasta or bread, choose whole-grain alternatives. Always look for *whole* wheat products because they have more fiber and nutrients. When a product is called "wheat," that does not necessarily mean it is made from whole wheat grains. If you're in doubt, check the label. If caramel coloring has been added, there's a good chance the actual wheat content in the product is low.

Whole wheat bread and pastas team with nutrients and fiber. *Oat bran* products (including oatmeal) help decrease the bad cholesterol in your blood system, thereby helping to prevent cancer and heart disease. The fiber in *wheat bran* also helps to prevent cancer by helping your body process your food. White bread, on the other hand, is almost devoid of fiber and natural nutrients. Try to eat natural grain products several times each day.

Reduce salt

We acquire our food tastes and cravings. If you take a newborn baby and never introduce salt into his or her diet, you reduce the chance that he or she will crave salt as an adult. Unfortunately, it wasn't until the 1950s when we discovered the harmful effects of too much salt. Because it may contribute to high blood pressure, we should try to limit our salt intake. (See Chapter Three for a more thorough discussion of high blood pressure in black men.)

In American culture, salt has become somewhat of a flavor-saver. If something tastes bad or bland, we put salt on it. Junk food such as peanuts, pretzels and potato chips contain a lot of salt.

To avoid salt, the first step is to remove your salt shaker from the table. Then, stock up on the many safe, healthy spices that can be used as salt substitutes. Try pepper, basil, oregano, garlic, Cajun spices, or spice preparations, such as Mrs. Dash.

Bacon	Luncheon meats
Baking powder	Monosodium glutamate (MSG)
Baking soda	Mustard
Beans (canned)	Olives
Bouillon (beef or chicken)	Pickles (dill or onion)
Bologna	Pig's feet (pickled)
Buttermilk (commercial)	Pizza
Canned meats (beef stew, chili)	Pot pies
Canned soups	Potato chips
Canned vegetables	Pretzels
Cheese	Salted nuts
Chitlins (pickled)	Saltines
Fast foods	Sauerkraut
Frozen prepared foods	Sausage
Hamburger	Seasonings†
Ham hock	Self-rising flour or meal
Hog maw (pickled)	Soda crackers
Hot dogs	Soy sauce
Instant grits	Steak sauces
Instant oatmeal	Tomato juice
Ketchup	TV dinners

†garlic salt, seasoning salt, onion salt, allspice, MSG, teriyaki, pre-mixed seasonings for meat, poultry and fish, lemon pepper

FIGURE 2F

Foods that are unusually high in salt.
Reprinted with permission of Macmillan Publishing Company from *High Blood Pressure* by Neil B. Shulman, Elijah Saunders, and W. Dallas Hall, copyright © 1987 by Neil B. Shulman, M.D., Elijah Saunders, M.D., and W. Dallas Hall, M.D.

Basil	Lemon juice
Celery seeds	Lime juice
Chili powder	Mint
Chives	Onion
Cinnamon	Onion powder
Curry	Oregano
Dill	Paprika
Flavoring extracts (vanilla, al- mond, walnut, peppermint, butter, lemon, etc.)	Pepper Pimento Soy sauce, low-sodium ("lite")*
Garlic	Wine, used in cooking (¼ cup)
Garlic powder	Worcestershire sauce
Hot pepper sauce	

*400 mg or more of sodium per exchange

FIGURE 2G

Seasonings that can replace salt.
Reprinted with permission from "Guidelines for the Use of Exchange Lists for Low-Sodium Meal Planning," copyright © 1989, American Diabetes Association, Inc.

Reduce your intake of fried food

When and if you do go to a fast food restaurant, try to order food that has not been fried. For example, many restaurants now offer broiled or baked chicken sandwiches, or salads as part of their menu. When you're cooking at home, use the same rule. Avoid eating fried food. Not only does frying require soaking the food in grease, the cooking process locks the fat inside the food. When you eat fried food, the fat is more likely to clog your arteries, adding inches to your waistline and putting you at higher risk of heart disease. Before biting into fried food, think of all that grease going straight for your heart, then decide if you *really* want to do that to your body.

Limit intake of red meat

Red meat, such as hamburgers and steaks, is filled with saturated fats and is high in "bad" cholesterol. Unfortunately, many of us have come to enjoy red meat as a regular part of our diet. Contrary to what was once taught, meat and potatoes do *not* make a healthy dinner. Many of us were told as children that red meat makes our bodies and muscles strong. After all, meat contains iron and protein, right?

Surprisingly, your body doesn't need as much protein as was once thought. Excess protein can actually decrease the absorption of other important nutrients in your body. You can get plenty of protein from healthy, delicious foods such as beans, tofu, fish, chicken (with the skin removed and *not* fried), low-fat dairy products and fruits, such as bananas.

By eating red meat, you may be substantially shortening your life, especially since that food has been closely linked to heart disease, the leading killer of black American men. If you can, give up red meat altogether. If you can't give it up, make a committed effort to eating meat only once in a while.

Eat fish instead of red meat

If you are looking for a healthy substitute for red meat, try fish. Fish is significantly lower in fat than red meat. Ask your medical professional for more information about the healthy benefits of eating fish. Be careful, however, to limit the amount of shellfish you eat (such as shrimp or lobster), since these tend to contain a lot of cholesterol.

There are many delicious kinds of fish. Experiment to find those that appeal to you most. If you're looking for a good substitute for red meat, swordfish and tuna steaks tend to be very dense, similar in texture to red meat, and delicious! Ask the attendant at your local fish market or the fish counter in your supermarket for ideas on ways to cook these and other fish. Just don't fry them or cook them with butter and oils, or coat them with fat, such as mayonnaise, butter or tartar sauce.

No more junk food

The junk food industry makes lots of money by making unhealthy foods seem very attractive. When buying pre-processed foods, do your research. Pretzels and crackers with less than two grams of fat per serving are excellent choices for snack food. Always check the sodium and fat content of other foods you buy as well. Most junk foods contain large amounts of salt, sugar and fat. A good rule is if it doesn't grow, don't eat it. If that doesn't work, at least think about how a certain food may be benefiting your body. Something such as soda pop, which hasn't been proven to cause cancer, offers your body absolutely nothing of value. If it's not helping, it may be part of the problem.

Fast food is one of the biggest contributors to the health problems facing the black community, especially in the South, where fast food mirrors the typical high-fat, high-salt Southerner's diet. Fast food is appealing everywhere because it's fast, readily available and affordable. Many people today have less time to prepare food for themselves and their families. As a result, we are all getting less good nutrition. There is a price to pay for speed and convenience.

When you purchase fast food, you're getting a lot more for your money than you realize. In addition to hamburgers and french fries, you're getting huge doses of cholesterol, fats, sodium and calories. Healthy American adults should consume no more than 67 grams of fat and 3,000 milligrams of sodium per day, according to the American Heart Association's dietary guidelines. If you go to Burger King and eat a Double Whopper with cheese, you've eaten 61 grams of fat and you're almost halfway to reaching your sodium limit. Throw in an order of french fries and you've surpassed your daily fat and sodium limit—in only one meal!

Say you like chicken more than hamburgers. You go to Kentucky Fried Chicken and order an Extra Crispy Chicken three-piece dinner, complete with mashed potatoes, gravy, coleslaw, and a biscuit. Maybe you think you've made the "healthy" choice because you've chosen chicken instead of red meat. Instead, you've just consumed 90.6 grams of fat in one meal alone—almost fifty percent more than your limit for the day. You've also consumed more than 1,400 calories, 3,049 milligrams of sodium (just over your allotment for the day) and 283 milligrams of cholesterol (300 is your daily maximum). After that one fast food meal, the only way you can keep within healthy dietary limits is not eating for the next couple of days. (We can all imagine how unhealthy, not to mention difficult, fasting can be!) As more blacks rely on fast food for their meals, it's no wonder that obesity is a growing problem in the black community.

Just because fast food restaurants are so prevalent and popular doesn't mean that they can't be bad. Fast food professionals—like everyone in business—are out to make money. If you buy unhealthy food, they will continue to sell it. Many employees of fast food restaurants will insist that their food is indeed healthy and getting healthier. It's true that some food chains now offer hamburgers that contain less fat, and even salads. Overall, however, most of the food served by these restaurants is extremely unhealthy.

Make careful choices. Before eating or drinking something, always ask yourself, "How is this helping my

Information is given per average serving				
Product	Calories	Sodium	Fat	Cholesterol
Potato chips (one ounce)	150	160 mg	10g	0
Pretzels (one ounce)	110	500 mg	1g	0
Peanuts (1.75 ounces)	290	140 mg	24g	0
Popcorn (3⅓ cups)	140	135 mg	8g	0
Corn chips (one ounce)	150	220 mg	10g	0

FIGURE 2H

Cholesterol, fat, sodium, and calorie content in junk food.
(taken from average products)

SNACK ON . . .

Air-popped popcorn with no butter, pretzels

Hard candy, jelly beans

Bagels, raisin toast, or English muffins with margarine or jelly

Low-fat cookies (such as fig bars, vanilla wafers, ginger snaps)

Fruits, vegetables

Fruit juices and drinks

Frozen yogurt, sherbet, ice pops

INSTEAD OF . . .

Popcorn with butter

Chocolate bars

Doughnuts, Danish pastry

Cake, cookies, brownies

Milk shakes, eggnogs, floats

Ice cream

FIGURE 21

Healthier snacking.
Reprinted from National Institute of Health: *Eat Right to Lower Your High Blood Cholesterol,* March 1992.

body?" If no answer comes to mind, ask yourself, "Is there something else I can eat or drink instead, which will give my body what it really needs?" If there is, it might be worth your while to go out of your way and make the healthy choice. A little extra effort now can save you a lot of suffering later. It's difficult to change lifelong eating habits. However, if you care enough about your health, you will find the motivation to modify your diet.

Drink lots of water and fresh fruit juice

The weight of our bodies is made up of more than 60 percent water. That's an awful lot! To maintain good health, we need to help our bodies maintain that proportion. You may be dehydrated more often than you realize. Without an adequate amount of water in our cells, our bodies have a tough time functioning. It's like expecting a car to keep on moving when it's almost out of gas!

The solution to helping our bodies maintain 60 percent of water is simple: drink water! Some say we should drink between eight and ten glasses of water each day. If you live in an area where your tap water is contaminated, you might want to research other options, such as drinking bottled water or using water filters. Some experts say that we can get away with drinking less water if we eat a lot of foods with a high water content, such as fruits and vegetables. Remember, however, that cooking removes the naturally high levels of water from these foods.

Drinking fresh fruit juice also boosts your body's water content. If you have a choice between eating an orange and drinking orange juice, it's usually healthier to choose the orange, because it contains fiber. If you're looking for something healthy to drink, however, 100 percent fruit juice is a great alternative to soda or fruit drinks. (Read labels carefully. While fruit drinks may claim to contain "real fruit juice," they often contain high levels of sugar and corn syrup, which decrease the fruit and vitamins you're receiving and increase your intake of sugar and empty calories.)

Not all drinks boost your water content, however. Drinks containing caffeine or alcohol can dehydrate water from your cells, reducing your body's water content. To be safe, get in the habit of drinking lots of water.

A word on diets

People who are overweight tend to have more heart problems than others because they generally don't get enough exercise—an important factor for a healthy heart and body. If you are carrying around extra weight, you're making your heart work harder. If you are already sedentary, you shouldn't put additional strain on your body with unnecessary weight.

Don't get lured into going on one of the quickie cure-all fad diets that are so popular today. By going on and off diets, you not only put your body in a dangerous habit of gaining and losing weight, you may also lose muscle and actually weaken your immune system and your ability to burn fat. Instead, change your eating habits and commit to a lifetime of healthy eating. You will lose weight gradually, naturally, and healthfully.

Try to follow the guidelines in this chapter every single day, for the rest of your life. Most importantly, limit your fat intake and eat lots of natural grain products, fresh fruits and vegetables. Remember, most fruits and vegetables contain no fat and actually equip your body with the fuel it needs to burn fat more efficiently. The best thing about fruits and vegetables is that you can eat a lot without risking gaining weight.

Also remember not to cover healthy foods with high-fat dressings or cheese, or with fat and cholesterol by frying them. Fried vegetables, such as french fries, can be particularly misleading. You may think you're doing something good for your body because you're eating vegetables, but, because they are fried, you are actually doing more harm than good. For seasonings, use lemon juice or spices. If you have to use a dressing, make sure it is low in fat or, better yet, fat-free. It may be a good idea to work with a physician, nurse, dietitian or health educator to design a medically sound diet that works for you. Your doctor can also help you to develop an exercise program that is personalized for your needs. Don't, however, be suckered into spending lots of money on quick cures. By following the guidelines outlined in this chapter, you are

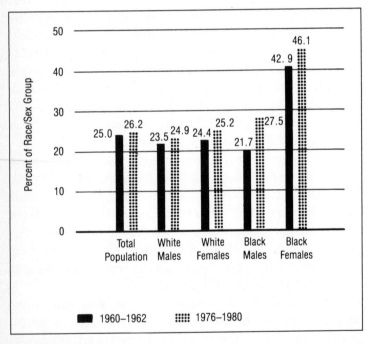

FIGURE 2J

Overweight trends by sex and race.
From *1993 Heart and Stroke Facts and Statistics*, copyright © 1993 American Heart Association. Reprinted with permission.

more likely to have a healthy body for life, not just a few months of thinness.

In addition to healthy food, exercise is very important when it comes to losing weight and maintaining good health. We should *all* make exercise a regular part of our lives. Later in this chapter, we'll discuss how to begin.

Stop smoking

Smoking is another bad habit that some of us use to relieve stress. Unfortunately, it's far from a cure. While it may seem like a "quick fix," the long-term consequences of smoking can be deadly. *Smoking is the single most preventable cause of premature death.* Smoking causes lung cancer and contributes to heart disease and stroke—the three leading killers of black men. If all black men were to avoid using tobacco, thousands of deaths could be avoided every year. If you smoke, stop. If you don't smoke, never start.

The Surgeon General has called nicotine an addicting drug for three reasons. First, when taken in small amounts, nicotine produces pleasurable feelings that make you want to smoke more. Second, smokers can become dependent on nicotine. They suffer both physical and psychological withdrawal symptoms when they stop smoking, such as nervousness, headaches and difficulty in sleeping. Third, nicotine is a drug that affects the chemistry of the brain and central nervous system, which explains how smoking affects one's mood and feelings. It is the addictive nature of smoking that makes it so difficult for many of us to quit.

If you're trying to stop smoking, you may have heard about alternative methods like cigarettes with less tar

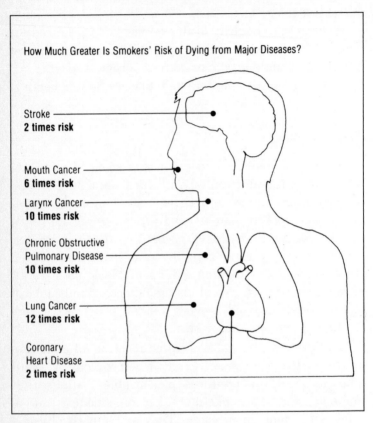

How Much Greater Is Smokers' Risk of Dying from Major Diseases?

Stroke —
2 times risk

Mouth Cancer —
6 times risk

Larynx Cancer —
10 times risk

Chronic Obstructive
Pulmonary Disease —
10 times risk

Lung Cancer —
12 times risk

Coronary
Heart Disease —
2 times risk

FIGURE 2K

Risks of smoking.
Reprinted from National Institute of Health, National Heart, Lung, and Blood Institute, "Nurses: Help Your Patients Stop Smoking," January 1993.

WITHDRAWAL SYMPTOM	THINGS YOU MIGHT DO
Craving for cigarettes	Do something else; take slow, deep breaths; tell yourself, "Don't do it."
Anxiety	Take slow, deep breaths; don't drink caffeine drinks; do other things.
Irritability	Walk; take slow, deep breaths; do other things.
Trouble sleeping	Don't drink caffeine drinks in evening; don't take naps during the day; imagine something relaxing like a favorite spot.
Lack of concentration	Do something else; take a walk.
Tiredness	Exercise; get plenty of rest.
Dizziness	Sit or lie down when needed; know it will pass.
Headaches	Relax; take mild pain medication as needed.
Coughing	Sip water.
Tightness in chest	Know it will pass.
Constipation	Drink lots of water; eat high-fiber foods such as vegetables and fruits.
Hunger	Eat well-balanced meals; eat low-calorie snacks; drink cold water.

FIGURE 2L

How to control the withdrawal symptoms of smoking.
Reprinted from National Institute of Health, National Heart, Lung, and Blood Institute, "Nurses: Help Your Patients Stop Smoking," January 1993.

and nicotine, chewing tobaccos and snuff. These are *not* safe alternatives. Studies show that menthol cigarettes may be even more dangerous to your health. About 28 percent of all U.S. cigarettes sold are menthol. Blacks smoke more menthol cigarettes than whites; about 76 percent of black cigarette smokers smoke menthol cigarettes compared with 23 percent of whites.

Menthol smokers can inhale more deeply or hold the smoke inside longer than smokers of nonmenthol cigarettes. This may be a reason why blacks, who actually smoke fewer cigarettes a day, are more likely than whites to die from smoking-related diseases—lung cancer, heart disease and stroke. Because smokeless tobacco contains nicotine (the same drug found in cigarettes), it is also harmful. In fact, snuff dippers take in over 10 times more cancer-causing substances (called nitrosamines) than cigarette smokers. These substances are absorbed through the lining of the mouth and can cause sores and white patches that often lead to cancer of the mouth.

Cigarette smoking can also be harmful to your arteries. If there is one thing that nearly all doctors agree on, it is that the most important controllable risk factor for cardiovascular disease is cigarette smoking. If you smoke, you have a 70 percent greater coronary heart disease death and stroke rate, and a twofold to fourfold greater risk of coronary heart disease and sudden death (the sudden, abrupt loss of heart function) than nonsmokers. In 1985, smoking was estimated to account for 21 percent of all coronary heart disease deaths and 40 percent of coronary heart disease deaths in people younger than age 65. Epidemiological studies have shown that your risk of death from heart disease will reduce greatly after you quit smoking. Some studies have shown a benefit within two years after quitting, while other studies have suggested that your risk of death will gradually decrease over a period of several years.

Nicotine damages the bodies not only of smokers but of nonsmokers as well. New studies indicate that passive smoking occurs when nonsmokers inhale the tobacco smoke of others, for example, sidestream smoke (the smoke that comes off the lit end of the cigarette). Sidestream smoke contains the same chemicals as the smoke inhaled by smokers and actually gives off larger amounts of cancer-causing substances.

Ask your doctor about available resources, support groups and other approaches, such as a nicotine patch, which may help you break your addiction to nicotine. Although quitting can be very difficult, chances are that once you experience what it is like to have smoke-free lungs, you'll agree it was worth the struggle.

Stop substance abuse

Smoking is not the only escape we use when we feel stressed. Some of us enjoy cocktails, beer, or drugs such as cocaine or marijuana. While these substances may make you feel good, the effect they have on your body is an entirely different story. These "feel good" potions may be killing you slowly. Drink after drink, drag after drag, your cells are dying, one by one, leading to disease and heartache for you and your loved ones.

Drinking alcohol, while legal for adults, is one of the most dangerous habits we can develop. While a drink every now and then may not hurt, alcohol is addictive and it is easy to become hooked. A leading killer of black men is cirrhosis of the liver, which is caused by heavy drinking. Because substance abuse is such a serious health problem, we have dedicated an entire chapter to this issue.

If substance abuse is of concern to you, read Chapter Ten carefully. Then, confide in your doctor. Together, you can fight your habit, whatever it may be. By working with a medical professional and making up your mind to change, good health can be yours again.

Exercise every day

Exercise programs can be seen on television stations across the country every morning. We see advertisements for exercise equipment, fashions and programs everywhere. No matter how commercial, the message is: exercise is good for you. Exercise reduces your risk of heart disease by decreasing the amount of cholesterol in your cardiovascular system, increases your HDL ("good") cholesterol, helps you maintain or lose weight, increases the strength of your heart muscle, increases the amount of enzymes in your body that burn fat, helps reduce stress, improves circulation, decreases blood pressure when it's elevated, decreases your percentage of body fat and increases the amount of muscle mass in your body. Regular exercise also helps your body burn fat, therefore promoting weight loss.

Aerobic exercise, such as walking, jogging, biking or swimming, uses a lot of energy and strengthens your heart and lungs. Regular aerobic exercise also improves circulation throughout your body and improves your body's ability to use oxygen. Exercise also builds energy levels, reduces stress and tension and helps you relax and sleep better.

Activity	Total Calories Used Per Hour*
Ballroom Dancing	125–310
Walking Slowly (2.5 mph)	210–230
Brisk Walking (4 mph)	250–345
Jogging (6 mph)	315–480
Cycling (9 mph)	315–480
Tennis	315–480
Basketball	480–625
Swimming	480–625
Cross Country Skiing	480–625

*Expenditure in calories by a 150-pound person.

FIGURE 2M

Energy expenditure for various sports.
Reprinted with permission of the Georgia Egg Commission: *Your Wellness Guide to a Healthy Lifestyle.*

It's never too late to start an exercise program. Just be sure to check with your doctor before you begin. Most physicians will gladly assist you in planning your personal fitness program. This is important because some exercises, such as weight lifting, can be quite strenuous and aren't a good option for everyone, especially those with disorders such as high blood pressure. Regardless of the exercise program you choose, make sure it's something you enjoy. Above all else, exercise should be fun.

According to the American Heart Association, your exercise program should ideally begin with a warmup period. The purpose is to prepare your body for the exercise to follow. The next phase of exercise, which is more vigorous, is the part that your heart and body will really appreciate because it will make your heart stronger and bring more oxygen into your body, both of which will make you feel better.

Exercise at least three times a week for a minimum of about 20 minutes each time. After you complete your exercise, always allow time to cool down. For example, after running, walk around for a little while so that your body cools down slowly.

Just don't overdo it. Take it slow and be patient with your body. As time goes by, you will find you'll be able to do more and more. Let this process happen naturally. Everyone's body is different. Listen to yours to learn when and when not to push yourself harder. Remember—exercise should be fun. This is important because, just like a healthy diet, exercise is a habit that should last for the rest of your life. Think of your exercise program as time to play—and enjoy it!

Reduce your stress

While exercise makes your immune system stronger, excess stress can make you more vulnerable to disease that may strike. Once you have a disease, stress can also weaken your body's ability to fight back. Blacks, in particular, suffer from a great deal of stress that often begins at childhood. Some say this is because of the racial discrimination we experience in social surroundings as well as work surroundings.

For example, think about how you feel when several white people cross the street when they see you walking toward them at night. Aren't you frustrated when a police officer stops your car to check your driver's license for no apparent reason? Or when you can't get a taxi to stop and pick you up? You're a black man. Our skin color often puts us in a disadvantageous position. Depending on where we live, events like these described may happen quite often. When they do, they can cause a lot of stress.

The real question is: Are you able to rise above this behavior pattern? Do you feel victimized and angry when you are mistreated because of the color of your skin? Or do you accept these insults as a challenge to prove your worth and integrity? Carefully watch the way your body reacts when you're in stressful situations. Your overall health and well-being are intricately tied to your state of mind. There are many ways to cope with the strains of daily living. Objective advice from a friend, counselor, minister, psychologist or psychiatrist may help. Meditation, exercise and entertainment are all ways to release tension after a stressful situation. Only you can take control of your own level of stress. To do this, you must become aware of the stress you are feeling by listening to your own mind and body.

When you realize you are experiencing excess stress, there are many techniques you can use to relax. Worrying too much over day-to-day problems can jeopardize your health. When you feel an excess amount of stress, do something about it.

Get involved in an activity that brings you pleasure. Usually, doing things that you do not enjoy brings on stress. To take your mind off a stress-causing situation, take a walk, get involved in a game, call a friend—do anything to remove yourself from the situation and relax and enjoy yourself. The situation may still be there when you come back, but the break will help you deal with it.

Take constructive action to make your life more relaxed. If your job seems to be a constant source of stress, try incorporating the above stress-reducing strategies into your daily life. Start a hobby or sport that you can look forward to doing at the end of a long working day. If you find yourself getting upset at work, make a conscious effort to think about things that make you happy or interests that you have outside of work. Take a short "coffee" or "bathroom" break, and instead, use the time to go for a brisk walk outside.

If you've tried all of these techniques for a period of time and none of them seem to be working, consider what options you have. Maybe it's time to consider changing jobs. If constant caretaking of children or an elderly person is stressful, ask a friend or family member to take over for a week. Whatever you do, don't attempt to relieve your stress by drinking, smoking, overeating or using drugs. While such habits may soothe your tension for a while, in the long run, they will add to it by harming your health and further complicating your life.

The *American Heritage Dictionary of the English Language* describes stress as "a mentally or emotionally disruptive or upsetting condition occurring in response to adverse external influences and capable of affecting physical health, usually characterized by increased heart rate, a rise in blood pressure, muscular tension, irritability and depression." In other words, stress, when out of control, can cause a great deal of emotional and physical damage. Learning to cope with these pressures is a key factor in maintaining a healthy lifestyle.

Get support

Most importantly, get your family and loved ones involved. If you are making changes in your lifestyle, it's important that those close to you understand and support the changes you are making. If your wife, mother or partner does most of the cooking in your family, have an honest, open conversation about your health and the changes you are making. You may want to recruit a friend or loved one into being your exercise partner. Making lifestyle changes is not always easy, but it is necessary for everyone. Involving your loved ones can be fun and can also bring additional closeness to your relationships.

There are also several support groups and organizations that can help you as you make changes. If you are looking to lose weight, you might want to investigate organizations like Overeaters Anonymous or Weight Watchers. If you're looking to reduce stress in your life, talk to someone at your local YMCA. They may be able to set up an exercise program for you, or recommend meditation or support groups that can help you work on specific issues of interest. Your doctor, dietitian, health educator or one of the professionals at your local health food store can also be invaluable resources when it comes to learning about organizations and programs in your area that can offer additional support.

A word on moderation

Regaining good health is a gradual process. Many of the lifestyle changes that we have discussed here may seem overwhelming or close to impossible. If you love red meat and can't imagine giving it up, don't go cold turkey.

Instead, just don't eat it as often. Take it slow. Remember, you are not alone. Thousands of black men just like you are grappling with the very same health issues. Look to your friends, family, physician and this book for support. Ultimately, however, the strength to change your lifestyle will come from within.

Good luck as you go forward. You can do it!

3

High Blood Pressure

Ned's story

"Who, me? High blood pressure? No way." That would have been Ned's response if anyone had asked him about having high blood pressure. That is, until the day his professor diagnosed him with hypertension during a health administration class.

Ned was 48 years old, well educated and conscientious about his health and appearance. He weighed just over 200 pounds, and the weight was well distributed over his six-foot frame. All in all, Ned had it made. In addition to being a handsome man with a good physique, he also had a good job and a great wife, Sharon, who supported him in everything he did. The couple had two sons, ages 13 and 11.

Ned was a successful hospital administrator at a large inner-city hospital. In fact, he was the first black administrator the hospital had ever had. After working in that capacity for over a year, Ned began taking night classes, working toward his doctorate degree. Sharon supported her husband's decision to further his education, although she saw less of him than usual and had to handle their two sons virtually alone.

One of Ned's assignments during his health administration course was to learn how to take blood pressure measurements. Ned, always willing, held up his hand when the professor asked for a volunteer. Besides, Ned was curious because he'd never really paid much attention to blood pressure readings. The professor took Ned's blood pressure three times; each reading was well above normal. Ned was surprised and more than a little concerned. The professor advised Ned that, although his blood pressure wasn't terribly high for a man his age, he should still have it checked by a doctor. Ned went home that night and told his wife about his blood pressure. She, too, was concerned, and they agreed to see their doctor as soon as possible.

After Ned's doctor had run a few tests and asked several background questions, he confirmed that Ned had high blood pressure. "But I don't feel sick," Ned said. "I feel great." The doctor explained that often people can have high blood pressure and not even know it. He also reassured the couple that high blood pressure is not a death sentence by any means. There are several things someone with high blood pressure can do to keep it under control.

Monroe's story

Monroe was a large man who worked as a butcher, just as his father and grandfather had before him. He was about thirty pounds overweight, with a smile that could stop you on the street and pull you into his butcher shop for laughs and a few pleasurable minutes.

Monroe's store, like a small-town barbershop, was the gathering place for people throughout the day. Monroe always had a pot of coffee on and a tray of sweets set out for the customers. At the end of his day, usually around six at night, Monroe would grab a few cuts of meat and head home.

Monroe liked all aspects of food—from preparation to cooking and eating. He especially liked salty foods. Whenever he brought meat home from the shop, he would cook big juicy steaks and then cover them with salt from the salt shaker. "You can never have enough salt," he used to say. "It improves the taste." Then he'd lick his lips jokingly. His wife used to tease him about it—it was an old joke between them. In Monroe and Cynthia's household, no meal was served without a salt shaker on the table.

One day, while Monroe was cutting ribs, he suddenly felt dizzy and weak. He set down his cleaver and leaned on the counter. The customer waiting for ribs was concerned. "Monroe, you look pale," he said uneasily. After about ten minutes, Monroe felt better and continued with the job at hand. That night, however, he told Cynthia about the incident. She asked him to go get a physical checkup. After all, it had been a couple of years since his last one. At first Monroe was against the idea, always picturing himself a strong, healthy man. After discussing *it further with his wife, however, he decided it was probably a good idea.*

High blood pressure is commonly called "hypertension" by doctors. By patients, it's called "the silent killer." That's because, like Ned and Monroe, you can have high blood pressure without even knowing it. Often, it sneaks up slowly. Maybe, like Monroe, you've always enjoyed eating salty foods. Or maybe, like Ned, you're under a lot of stress. Without even knowing it, you may be leading a lifestyle destined for tragedy. Unless, of course, you're willing to make a change.

If you have high blood pressure, you should know that it's very common. Hypertension can be caused by your lifestyle, a predisposition in your genes, or both. If someone in your family had high blood pressure, keep a close eye on your own. You may be at increased risk. But whether you have been diagnosed with hypertension or you haven't, it's important for you and your family to know how this disease can be prevented and treated.

What is high blood pressure?

Blood pressure is the pressure of blood against the walls of your blood vessels—especially your arteries. Your heart pumps blood through your arteries with varying degrees of force. For example, certain types of exercises, such as lifting weights, cause your heart to pump harder and blood vessels to tighten, resulting in more pressure inside your blood vessels.[1]

There is a difference between hypertension, which is a health disorder, and occasional elevated blood pressure caused by normal physiological reactions. When you are participating in a strenuous activity or feeling emotional stress, such as excitement or anger, your blood pressure can rise. However, this does not necessarily mean you have high blood pressure or hypertension. Do you remember ever being so frightened that you thought your heart would jump out of your chest? Maybe this happened when you were nervous, such as during a job interview or review. Although your blood pressure measurement may be high during activities like these, it quickly returns to normal. If you have high blood pressure or hypertension, on the other hand, your blood pressure stays constantly above what is considered normal.

Why are blacks at greater risk?

Black males are 40 percent more likely to suffer from high blood pressure than white males, and we usually suffer more serious complications, such as kidney failure. Approximately 28 percent of all people on kidney dialysis machines are black. Meanwhile, as a group, we only make up 12 percent of the population! High blood pressure kills black men 15.5 times more often than it does white men, and one of four blacks has high blood pressure. (Hypertension is more common among younger men than women; however in middle age, more women than men have hypertension. This may be due to the effect of women going through menopause.)

Why are blacks more likely to suffer from high blood pressure than others? This question is tough to answer, because the cause of 95 percent of all hypertension cases has not yet been proven. However, one characteristic that hypertensive patients seem to have in common is "too much"—too much salt in the diet, too much stress, too

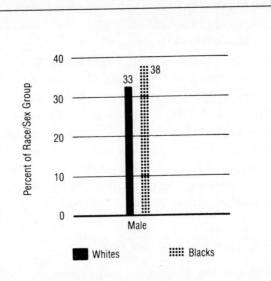

Hypertensives are defined as persons with a systolic level ≥140 and/or a diastolic level ≥90 or who report using antihypertensive medication. (Your systolic blood level is the number that appears on the top of the fraction that represents your blood pressure. Your diastolic level is the number that appears on the bottom. A more detailed explanation of what these numbers represent appears later in this chapter.)

FIGURE 3A

Rates of hypertension for men adjusted by age.
Reprinted with permission of the American Heart Association, *1993 Heart and Stroke Facts and Statistics,* copyright © 1992, American Heart Association.

much weight, too much alcohol. High blood pressure may be caused by one of these factors or a combination of several of them.

Do we have an inherited kidney defect?

In one study, researchers suggested that blacks may have inherited a kidney defect that limits their ability to process sodium, an element found in salt. If this theory is correct, people with the kidney defect would not be able to properly handle salt already in their bodies, let alone any additional salt they add through diet. If you have inherited this condition, this means that any salt in your food may cause your blood pressure to rise, putting you at a high risk for hypertension.[2]

Did it really all start with slavery?

Dr. Clarence Grimm of Drew Medical Center in Los Angeles offers another theory. Grimm says that when slave trading was practiced with African natives, the physical demands of the ocean voyage were very great. Many slaves died of dehydration or loss of water in their body tissues. Salt is necessary to hold water in your tissues; therefore, according to Grimm, only the best "salt savers" survived. While saving salt and retaining fluid was a boon on a voyage with little fresh water, the same characteristic may actually be harmful under normal conditions, because it makes you more susceptible to high blood pressure. Since the tendency toward high blood pressure is often hereditary, Grimm suggests that the first Americanized "salt savers" passed their strong tendency toward "salt saving" to future generations.[3] You can take this with a grain of salt!

City living can lead to hypertension

Several studies also show that hypertension increases with the stress of urbanization. In 1984, Neil Poulter studied a tribe in Kenya that migrated to the city of Nairobi. He was able to study their blood pressures before and after the migration. Overall, the blood pressures of the tribe members increased. Later, the tribe was forced to flee the city due to political unrest. After the tribe members returned to a rural setting, Poulter saw that their blood pressures returned to their original low levels.

Ironically, our African ancestors were almost hypertension-free. However, as they moved away from their tribal villages to cities, high blood pressure became more common. This could be due to several factors, such as overcrowding, poverty, increased salt intake, poor eating habits leading to weight gain, or stress from political or racial discrimination. Whatever the reason, something has caused the blood pressure of formerly unaffected Africans to rise.

Discrimination causes stress

Some researchers, such as Michael Klag, whose study was published in the *Journal of the American Medical Association (JAMA)*, report that darker skin color itself can be a cause of stress that can lead to high blood pressure. Many dark black men who struggle daily to climb the socioeconomic ladder encounter complications because of racial barriers. These include stagnant job level, racism in the workplace, and sometimes "guilt by color." For example, when something goes wrong or winds up missing from the office, a black male may be more likely to be suspected and accused than his white coworkers. Understandably, this can be very frustrating, especially if it happens often. This constant level of frustration may contribute to high blood pressure.[4]

Two types of hypertension

There are two types of hypertension. The first, known as "essential hypertension," accounts for approximately 95 percent of all high blood pressure cases. "Essential hypertension" refers to those cases that occur due to unknown reasons. While research has shown a link between certain factors and hypertension, no direct causal relationship has been proven. Both Monroe and Ned were diagnosed with "essential hypertension."

"Secondary hypertension" accounts for the other five percent of all high blood pressure cases. "Secondary hypertension" is caused by specific abnormalities such as tumors, kidney disease, the blockage of certain arteries (such as kidney artery), or high levels of certain substances in your blood, such as cocaine. Cocaine and crack have recently become established as common causes of secondary hypertension. (For more information about drug and substance abuse, see Chapter Ten.) Also, when secondary hypertension has been caused by a tumor releasing an adrenaline-type substance, it can sometimes be corrected by surgery.

Now, let's look again at the cases of Ned and Monroe.

Ned and Monroe react to their diagnoses

Ned, upon learning of his condition, was anxious to know why he developed high blood pressure. Since he and his wife had decided to treat the disorder aggressively rather than sit back and let the disorder run its course, it was important for him to know its origin. He read all the latest studies and articles concerning high blood pressure and talked to his doctor extensively. He and his wife also looked into his family tree, to see if his high blood pressure could possibly be genetic.

They learned that some of Ned's family members were also living with the disease. "My uncle is an insurance broker," said Ned. "He travels a lot and eats out often. He knows better, but admits he doesn't watch his diet even though he takes his medicine regularly without fail.

"A cousin of mine didn't discover she had high blood pressure until she became pregnant," Ned continued. "The doctors watched her carefully during the delivery and she has been on medication ever since. She is very careful about her diet."

By looking at their own diets, Ned and Sharon learned that Ned regularly consumed too much sodium (found primarily in salt), a factor that can contribute heavily to the development of the disease.

When Monroe visited his doctor, he learned that his blood pressure was at a dangerous level. After answering a lot of questions, Monroe discovered that his lifestyle fit the classic profile of a hypertension candidate. Several factors had contributed to his high blood pressure. Heredity, for one. Like Ned, Monroe had a family history of high blood pressure. Of all the factors, however, Monroe's diet was probably the biggest contributor to his condition. Monroe admitted to his doctor that he had a habit of always salting his food before he even tasted it.

In addition, Monroe had many bad eating habits, such as his love of red meat and peanuts. Because he had been eating fat-filled foods like these throughout his entire life, Monroe learned that he was also a high-risk candidate for heart disease (see Chapter Four). This complicated his condition even further.

The doctor talked to Monroe and Cynthia for a long time, explaining the benefits of good diet and exercise. Monroe never was one to exercise, preferring to spend his spare time in deep conversation with customers. The couple listened to the doctor intently and, upon leaving the office, stopped by their local pharmacy to fill Monroe's new prescription. Monroe took his medicine for hypertension every day, but was unwilling to change his diet. Cynthia tried to convince her husband to eat more healthy foods, without success.

How can I prevent high blood pressure?

In Chapter Two, we discussed many ways to prevent disease. Although no studies have proven a single cause of "essential" hypertension, several factors have been closely linked to preventing this condition from developing into fatal consequences, such as heart attack or stroke.

Limit salt in your diet

Studies show that too much salt in the diet is closely associated with hypertension. To prevent and treat high blood pressure, it's very important to reduce your salt intake. For more information about salty foods to avoid and how to improve your diet, see Chapter Two.

Reduce stress

A number of different factors have been associated with high blood pressure. Stress is one. Like Ned, many of us lead active, hectic lives. While we may find our busy lives fulfilling, constantly putting ourselves in situations that make us tense puts huge amounts of pressure on ourselves and our circulatory systems. We should all make a conscious effort to reduce our stress levels, especially if someone in our family has already had high blood pressure, meaning we may be at increased risk. (More information about stress reduction is also included in Chapter Two.)

Increase your potassium intake

When it comes to preventing hypertension, it's also important to make sure you are getting enough potassium in your diet. Research shows a link between low potassium intake and high blood pressure. Many studies show that blacks in the United States consume less potassium than whites. One reason for this may be the fact that overall, blacks eat less fresh fruit than whites. Both fresh fruits and vegetables contain high levels of potassium. However, remember—if you overcook vegetables, you lose much of the potassium and vitamins that these foods offer. Also, if you choose prune juice as a source of potassium, it's important for you to realize that prunes are also a laxative. If you notice your stools getting loose, choose another potassium source instead.

Try to increase your intake of potassium naturally through foods, if you can. Just don't overdo it. No study has proven that taking potassium supplements will necessarily lower your blood pressure, so get your doctor's approval before taking this route. In fact, high potassium levels can be dangerous if you have an illness such as kidney disease, so you'll want to be especially careful if this pertains to you.

Item	Amount	Milliequivalents of Potassium	Calories	Milligrams of Sodium‡
Prune juice*	1 glass†	15.1	193	5
Tomato juice	1 glass	13.7	48	480
Cantaloupe	One-half	12.8	60	24
Potato (baked)	One medium	12.8	95	4
Grapefruit juice	1 glass	11.8	108	3
Orange juice	1 glass	10.7	120	3
Milk (skim)	1 glass	10.5	89	128
Raisins	⅓ cup	10.4	153	14
Milk (whole)	1 glass	9.5	150	120
Banana	One (6″)	9.5	85	1
Pineapple juice	1 glass	9.2	128	<1
Tomato	One medium	8.1	29	5
Orange	One medium	8.0	71	2
Pear	One medium	6.7	122	4
Apple juice	1 glass	6.2	120	8
Peach	One medium	5.2	38	1
Apple	One medium	4.2	87	1
Grapefruit	One-half	3.5	41	1
Black coffee	1 cup	2.2	2	1

*All juice values are as canned, unsweetened

†1 glass = 8 ounces

‡Remember, the recommended daily limit for sodium intake is 3000 milligrams.

FIGURE 3B

Potassium-rich foods.
Reprinted with permission of Macmillan Publishing Company, from *High Blood Pressure* by Neil B. Shulman, Elijah Saunders, and W. Dallas Hall, copyright © 1987 by Neil B. Shulman, M.D., Elijah Saunders, M.D., and W. Dallas Hall, M.D.

Increase your calcium intake

Some researchers have also suggested that low levels of calcium in your diet may contribute to hypertension. However, this is still under debate.

	mg calcium
MILK GROUP	
Buttermilk, 1 cup	285
Cheese, American 1 oz.	174
Cheese, Cheddar, 1 oz.	204
Cheese, Ricotta, Part Skim (4 oz.)	337
Cheese, Swiss, 1 oz.	272
Ice Cream, vanilla, ½ cup	88
Milk, 1 cup	291
Milk, lowfat (2%), 1 cup	297
Milk, skim, 1 cup	302
Yogurt, fruit, lowfat, 1 cup	345
Yogurt, plain, lowfat, 1 cup	415
MEAT GROUP	
Beans, dried, cooked, 1 cup	90
Oysters, raw, 7–9	113
Salmon, canned with bones, 3 oz.	167
Sardines, with bones, 3 oz.	372
Shrimp, canned, 3 oz.	99
FRUIT-VEGETABLE GROUP	
Beet Greens, ½ cup	72
Bokchoy, ½ cup	126
Broccoli, stalk, ½ cup	68

	mg calcium
Collards, from raw, ½ cup	179
Collards, from frozen, ½ cup	149
Kale, from raw, ½ cup	103
Kale, from frozen, ½ cup	79
Mustard Greens, ½ cup	97
Spinach, ½ cup	84
GRAIN GROUP	
Cornbread, 2½ by 2½ by 1½ inches	94
Pancakes, 4-inch diameter, 2	116
Waffles, 7-inch diameter	179

FIGURE 3C

Selected calcium-rich food sources.
Reprinted with permission from the American Dairy Association booklet *Calcium-Rich Everyday Foods.*

Avoid licorice and chewing tobacco

In some cases, licorice and chewing tobacco can cause high blood pressure because these substances may contain a steroidlike compound that stimulates your kidneys to hold on to sodium. This compound also causes your body to hold onto fluids, which can elevate your blood pressure. So if you are prone to high blood pressure, it's best to avoid licorice and chewing tobacco.[5]

Prevent and treat obesity

Excess weight puts a strain on your heart as well as your body. High blood pressure is more common in obese people than in people with normal body weight. If you know you are prone to high blood pressure, it would be especially wise for you to keep your weight at the ideal amount for your height and body frame. If you think you should lose weight, consult your doctor. Then, reread Chapter Two for tips on how to begin.

How do I know if I have hypertension?

If you experience sudden temporary blindness, chest pain, dizziness or severe pounding headaches, see a doctor immediately, since these can be symptoms of severe high blood pressure. Nosebleeds, while common among people with normal blood pressure levels, can also be a sign of dangerously high blood pressure. If you're experiencing any of these symptoms, get your blood pressure checked immediately.

Even if you're not experiencing these symptoms, it's still important to monitor your blood pressure regularly. Like Ned, many people aren't aware they have high blood pressure. If left undetected and untreated, hypertension can surprise you in the form of a heart attack, stroke, kidney failure or blindness. (See Chapter Four for more information about heart disease.) To find out if you need to take precautions against these tragedies, have a health professional check your blood pressure. Or you can check it yourself.

Taking your blood pressure

You have two options: You can take your own blood pressure or have someone else take it. If you decide to take it, you need a blood pressure kit. The kit will con-

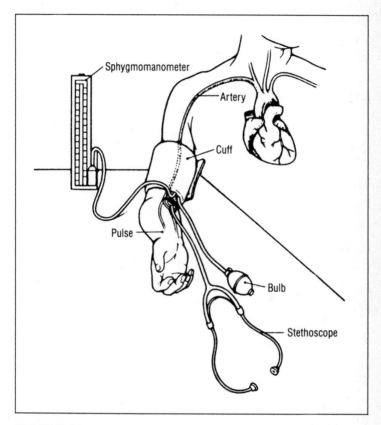

FIGURE 3D

How blood pressure is measured.
Reprinted with permission of the Macmillan Publishing Company, from *High Blood Pressure* by Neil B. Shulman, Elijah Saunders, and W. Dallas Hall, copyright © 1987 by Neil B. Shulman, M.D., Elijah Saunders, M.D., and W. Dallas Hall, M.D.

tain an arm cuff with a pressure gauge attached to it
(sphygmomanometer) and a listening device (stethoscope). You'll need to purchase a cuff that is the correct
width for your arm. Large widths are necessary if the
circumference of your upper arm is more than 13 inches.
This kit can be purchased at most pharmacies for about
$30. You can also purchase a more expensive blood pres-
sure kit that is totally automated.

Before you take your blood pressure, make sure you
are relaxed and have been sitting down for at least five
minutes.

Then—

1. Locate your pulse in the bend of your elbow with
   your finger.
2. Wrap the cuff around your upper arm, leaving about
   one inch between the bottom of the cuff and the bend
   of your elbow. Be sure that nothing is caught under
   the cuff, such as your clothing, since this may affect
   the reading.
3. Hold the rubber bulb so that the screw lies between
   your thumb and first finger. Inflate the cuff by squeez-
   ing the rubber bulb until you can no longer feel your
   pulse beat in your wrist. Write down the number on
   the gauge at this point.
4. Turn the screw toward you (to the right), releasing
   the pressure out of the cuff until the gauge reads zero.
5. Add 30 to the first number you wrote down and pump
   up the cuff until the gauge reads this number.
6. Place the stethoscope directly over the main artery of
   your arm (brachial artery).
7. Releasing the air on the gauge, listen for the first tapping sound. When you hear it, note the number on the

gauge. This is the systolic pressure, the top number of
your blood pressure reading.

8. The number on the gauge at the last sound or tapping
noise you hear is the diastolic pressure, the bottom
number of your blood pressure.[6]

If you have a hearing impairment, you may not be able
to hear the tapping sounds through the stethoscope. Your
doctor or a nurse should be able to instruct you in your
blood pressure measurement and verify the accuracy of
your equipment by checking your readings with their
own.

What happens when my blood pressure is taken?

When the cuff is wrapped around your upper arm and
inflated, the air pressure in the cuff pushes against the
main artery of your arm and nearby bone. This stops
your flow of blood. When the pressure is released, your
blood flows freely again, making a "whooshing" sound
through the narrowed artery. The number on the gauge
when this sound is made is the systolic pressure. A normal blood pressure reading is less than 130/85, the systolic pressure measurement being the top number and
diastolic being the bottom number. When your blood flow
finally evens out and your blood vessel is no longer narrowed, the sound disappears. The number on the gauge at
the last sound you will hear will be the diastolic pressure.
Except in extreme cases, the lower your blood pressure
is, the better off you are. The higher your blood pressure,
the greater risk you run of having complications.

If you decide to have someone else take your blood
pressure, you have several options. Any medical professional—including health clinic employees, nurses, health

**CLASSIFICATION OF BLOOD PRESSURE FOR ADULTS
AGE 18 YEARS AND OLDER***

Category	Systolic (mm Hg)	Diastolic (mm Hg)
Normal†	<130	<85
High normal	130–139	85–89
Hypertension**		
STAGE 1 (mild)	140–159	90–99
STAGE 2 (Moderate)	160–179	100–109
STAGE 3 (Severe)	180–209	110–119
STAGE 4 (Very Severe)	≥210	≥120

* Not taking antihypertensive drugs and not acutely ill. When systolic and diastolic pressures fall into different categories, the higher category should be selected to classify the individual's blood pressure status. For instance, 160/92 mm Hg should be classified as Stage 2, and 180/120 mm Hg should be classified as Stage 4. Isolated systolic hypertension (ISH) is defined as SBP≥140 mm Hg and DBP <90 mm Hg and staged appropriately (e.g., 170/85 mm Hg is defined as Stage 2 ISH).

† Optimal blood pressure with respect to cardiovascular risk is SBP<120 mm Hg and DBP <80 mm Hg. However, unusually low readings should be evaluated for clinical significance.

** Based on the average of two or more readings taken at each of two or more visits following an initial screening.

Note: In addition to classifying stages of hypertension based on average blood pressure levels, the clinician should specify presence or absence of target-organ disease and additional risk factors. For example, a patient with diabetes and a blood pressure of 142/94 mm Hg plus an enlarged left heart muscle (left ventricular hypertrophy) should be classified as "Stage 1 hypertension with target-organ disease (left ventricular hypertrophy) and with another major risk factor (diabetes)." This specificity is important for risk classification and management.

FIGURE 3E

Severity of high blood pressure.
Reprinted from the Fifth Report of the Joint National Committee on Detection, Evaluation, and Treatment of High Blood Pressure, from the National Institute of Health, Heart, Lung, and Blood Institute, NIH publication No. 93-1008, January 1993.

educators, doctors, dentists, and pharmacists—should be able to take your blood pressure reading. It's always a good idea to ask your doctor to take your blood pressure whenever you visit, even if you are there for another reason. Let your doctor or health care professional know that you would like your blood pressure checked on a regular basis. They can help find an inexpensive or even free way to keep your pressure checked regularly.

An adult's blood pressure is ideal when it is less than 130/85, considered to be a "normal" blood pressure. If your blood pressure is within this range, it is safe to have it checked every other year until you reach age 40. If you are older than 40 and/or your blood pressure is higher than 130/85, you should get a regular checkup done twice a year.

Ned, Monroe and stress

When Ned reflected on his lifestyle, in search of clues to why he had high blood pressure, he found that stress was a factor. This stress came from his job position and, more recently, the additional pressure of taking night classes after work. When Ned became a hospital administrator, it was a big deal. However, his job, even with all its glory, had its drawbacks. Ned worked long hours to keep up with the mountain of paperwork that gathered on his desk weekly.

Sometimes, against his wife's wishes, he still works weekends. "He always says, 'If I work late this one night, I'll be caught up,' or, 'Just this one weekend and then never again,'" said his wife. Ned admits the workload has, indeed, been heavy. He can tell this by the effect it has been having on his everyday life. Frequent head-aches, loss of appetite, sleeplessness—all became part of Ned's daily routine. The long hours coupled with the re-sponsibility of supervising an entire section of the hos-pital had a direct effect on Ned's stress level. Fortunately, he has learned to alleviate stress buildup through exercise.

"Sharon and I don't have all the answers," said Ned. "But we're both determined to do everything possible to keep my disease under control. It helps when you have support from your family. This isn't something you can do alone."

Monroe's Eating Habits

In Monroe's search for the cause of his high blood pres-sure, in contrast to Ned's, stress was nowhere near the top of the list. Diet and obesity were Monroe's number-one and number-two risk factors.

Although Monroe knew his eating habits were not great, he was not willing to change them. Despite Cyn-thia's efforts, she couldn't be with him every minute of every day to monitor his lifestyle. Much to his dismay, she took over cooking at home to ensure that healthy foods were prepared. She still let him cook an occasional steak, but tried to center meals around chicken and fish prepared by baking or broiling. She refused to use salt when cooking, substituting for it with a variety of spices and seasoning. When Monroe was on his own, however, the only right thing he did was take his medicine. Since his wife wouldn't let him eat salty food at home, he started going to fast food restaurants every day for lunch. Because he wasn't willing to take control of his own health, he began gaining even more weight.

What can happen if I don't treat my hypertension?

If you have been diagnosed with high blood pressure and, like Monroe, decide not to make important lifestyle changes, the consequences can be deadly.

Your risk of having a stroke increases

Left untreated, high blood pressure can cause strokes. While the exact reason for this is not known, it seems that high blood pressure injures your arterial walls and allows plaques (fat and cholesterol buildup) to attach to the scarring. When high blood pressure goes unchecked, it can sometimes cause enough buildup of fatty deposits and pressure to completely block your arteries. When this blockage occurs in an artery that supplies your brain with blood, a stroke may occur. We discuss strokes further in Chapter Four. According to the Office of Minority Health, blacks have strokes twice as often as whites. Black men are also almost twice as likely to die from stroke as white men.

You are at greater risk of kidney disease

Uncontrolled high blood pressure can also damage your kidneys. When your kidneys are damaged, their ability to rid your body of wastes becomes impaired, which can result in a whole host of diseases and disorders related to kidney malfunction. See Chapter Eight for more detailed information on kidney or renal failure.

You may develop heart disease

High blood pressure contributes to heart disease. As the amount of pressure increases in your arteries, your

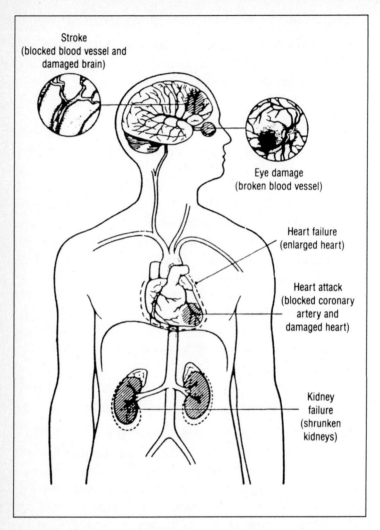

FIGURE 3F

Complications of high blood pressure.
Reprinted with permission of Macmillan Publishing Company, from *High Blood Pressure* by Neil B. Shulman, Elijah Saunders, and W. Dallas Hall, copyright © 1987 by Neil B. Shulman, M.D., Elijah Saunders, M.D., and W. Dallas Hall, M.D.

heart has to work harder to circulate blood throughout your body. The harder your heart works, the more your heart muscle builds and enlarges, making it less efficient. Also, the blood vessels that supply blood to your heart itself, the coronary arteries, may become blocked, resulting in death of heart tissue (heart attack). For more detailed information on heart disease, see Chapter Four.

How can I treat my high blood pressure?

Unfortunately, black males are notorious for not seeking and continuing treatment. Approximately 50 percent of black men with high blood pressure drop out of treatment in the first year. One-third of those who stay under medical care do not take their prescribed medicine regularly enough to achieve adequate blood pressure reduction. This may be one reason why so many more black men than white men die of complications from high blood pressure.

Once you have complications from high blood pressure, the cost can rocket from about $30 a month for medication to control high blood pressure to around $35,000 a year for dialysis treatment of a failed kidney. In other words, you will save yourself a lot of money and suffering by controlling your blood pressure with medication.

Exercise

Exercise, exercise, exercise. Regular exercise improves circulation throughout your body and enhances your body's ability to use oxygen. Exercise also increases your energy level, reduces stress and tension, helps you lose weight and makes it easier for you to relax and sleep.

It is never too late to start an exercise program. Before you begin, ask your doctor for advice, especially if you have already been diagnosed with high blood pressure, because certain types of exercise, such as weight-lifting, may be dangerous. For more information about how to begin your own personalized exercise program, see Chapter Two.

Limit your alcohol intake

If you're already hypertensive, alcohol consumption makes your disorder more difficult to control and can get in the way of blood pressure medication. Limit your alcohol intake. Ideally, you should avoid it altogether. However, if you choose to drink alcohol, use the rule of moderation. Try to limit your daily intake to no more than one or two drinks (a drink being a 6-ounce glass of wine, an 8-ounce glass of beer, or a 1-ounce shot of hard liquor).

Take your high blood pressure medication

Your doctor will tell you which medications, if any, you should take if you are diagnosed with high blood pressure. But it is up to you to ask questions. Many high blood pressure medications can cause side effects. You and your doctor should choose one that will work best for you.

Hypertension medication

When your doctor prescribes new medication, ask him or her for free samples. That way, if you develop an unpleasant side effect, you have not wasted money by purchasing an entire prescription. There are many hypertension medications on the market today. Make sure you are taking one that best suits your needs. After all, once you have high blood pressure, you will usually have it for the rest of your life, and you'll need to continue taking medication.

Impotence is one side effect that prevents some men from staying on blood pressure medication. It is important to remember that impotence is a rare side effect of high blood pressure medication, and recent advances have been made in high blood pressure medication that allow the disorder to be treated without causing this side effect. To find out if impotence is a possible side effect of your medication, consult the list of high blood pressure medications in Figure 3G. If you are currently using a prescription that may cause impotence and you suffer from this, ask your doctor about possibly changing your prescription.[7]

No matter what, do not stop taking your high blood pressure medication without your doctor's consent, even if you're feeling great. Remember, hypertension is a "silent killer" that won't think twice about doing you in.

Remember to take your medication

So you're forgetful? Afraid you can't remember to take your pills? Here are some suggestions that may help you.

1. Place your pills or capsules where you will notice them when doing a daily task, such as brushing your teeth.
2. Keep your pills in separate containers that are labeled with the time you should take them, such as at breakfast, lunch, dinner, or at bedtime.

Brand or Trade Name	Generic Name	Examples of Bothersome Side Effects
Accupril	quinapril	cough, rash
Adalat	nifedipine	headache, swelling of legs
Aldomet	methyldopa	sleepiness, impotence, hepatitis
Altace	ramipril	cough, rash
Apresoline	hydralazine	headaches, pounding heart, lupus erythematosus
Blocadren	timolol	fatigue, shortness of breath
Bumex	bumetanide	weak muscles, frequent urination, gout
Calan	verapamil	constipation, dizziness
Capoten	captopril	cough, rash
Cardene	nicardipine	headache, swelling of legs
Cardizem	diltiazem	headache, dizziness
Cardura	doxazosin	dizziness
Catapres	clonidine	sleepiness, dry mouth
Corgard	nadalol	fatigue, shortness of breath, numb hands
Dyazide	†	frequent urination, gout
DynaCirc	isradipine	headache, swelling of legs
Esidrix	hydrochlorothiazide	weak muscles, frequent urination, gout
Hygroton	chlorthalidone	weak muscles, frequent urination, gout
Hylorel	guanadrel	dizziness, passing out
Hytrin	terazosin	dizziness
Inderal	propranolol	fatigue, shortness of breath, sleep disturbance, numb hands
Ismelin	guanethidine	dizziness, passing out, impotence

Brand or Trade Name	Generic Name	Examples of Bothersome Side Effects
Isoptin	verapamil	constipation, dizziness
Kerlone	betaxolol	fatigue, shortness of breath, numb hands
Lasix	furosemide	weak muscles, frequent urination, gout
Levatol	penbutalol	fatigue, shortness of breath, numb hands
Loniten	minoxidil	swelling of legs, excess hair growth
Lopressor	metoprolol	fatigue, sleep disturbance
Lotensin	benazepril	cough, rash
Lozol	metolazone	weak muscles, frequent urination, gout
Maxzide	†	frequent urination, gout
Minipress	prazosin	dizziness, irregular heartbeat
Monopril	fosinopril	cough, rash
Naturetin	bendroflumethiazide	weak muscles, frequent urination, gout
Normodyne	labetalol	fatigue, dizziness, tingling scalp
Norvasc	amlodipine	headache, swelling of legs
Plendil	felodipine	headache, swelling of legs
Prinivil	lisinopril	cough, rash
Procardia	nifedipine	headache, swelling of legs

† A combination type HTN drug—a diuretic containing hydrochlorothiazide and triamterene

FIGURE 3G

Side effects of high blood pressure medication.
Reprinted with permission of Macmillan Publishing Company, from *High Blood Pressure* by Neil B. Shulman, Elijah Saunders, and W. Dallas Hall, copyright © 1987 by Neil B. Shulman, M.D., Elijah Saunders, M.D., and W. Dallas Hall, M.D.

3. Wear a watch with an alarm that rings when you need to take your medication.
4. Mark your calendar every time you take your medicine.
5. At the beginning of each day, set out the pills you need to take.
6. Keep extra pills handy, in case you run out before your next visit to the doctor.
7. If you are going out for the day, or on vacation, remember to pack/take your medication with you.

Ned, Monroe and exercise

Ned isn't overweight, but he exercises several days a week, sometimes with Sharon, sometimes by himself. He runs three days a week—sometimes before work and sometimes after, depending on his schedule. He also plays basketball with his friends at least two times a week. He says that the activity seems to reduce his stress level and make him feel better. "It's a lot easier to face the day after a vigorous walk or jog," Ned said. "I also find that running after work is a good time to reflect on my day."

Monroe's story took a different turn. The exercise program suggested by his doctor never got farther than the walk to the bakery.

Conclusion

Don't let yourself become a victim of your condition, like Monroe. If you were able to identify with any of the risks mentioned in this chapter, act now. Although black males seem to be more prone to hypertension than other people, you don't have to become the next statistic. Take a long, hard look at your lifestyle. It is never too late to learn from stories like those of Ned and Monroe.

Monroe's health continues to fail. Although he still takes his medication, he takes no responsibility for his treatment. Instead of taking control, Monroe is becoming a victim of his high blood pressure.

Ned, on the other hand, took an aggressive attitude toward controlling his high blood pressure. As a result, today he enjoys a healthy lifestyle. The only reminder he has of his condition is his high blood pressure medicine, which he takes every day. Because he was willing to make changes in his lifestyle, Ned has found new levels of fulfillment by taking personal responsibility for his own health and relying on his family and friends for support.

Resources

American Red Cross
2025 E Street N.W.
Washington, DC 20009
(202) 728-6400

(Contact your local chapter for services provided by the American Red Cross related to high blood pressure.)

High Blood Pressure Information Center
PO Box 30105
Bethesda, MD 20824-0105
(301) 251-1222

(The Center gives patient information and referrals for programs in your local area.)

International Society on Hypertension in Blacks
2045 Manchester Street
Atlanta, GA 30324-4110
(404) 875-6263

(The Society provides materials on conferences, workshops and research, as well as patient education brochures. Membership is available.)

National Kidney Foundation
30 East 33rd Street
New York, NY 10016
(212) 889-2210

(The Foundation provides a catalog that lists all materials available through your local kidney foundation office.)

US Pharmacopoeial Convention, Inc.
12601 Twin Brook Parkway
Rockville, MD 20852
(301) 881-0666

(The Convention distributes the book "About Your High Blood Pressure Medicines" at a cost of $7.50 each.)

◆

4

Heart Disease and Stroke

SECTION ONE:
HEART DISEASE

Claude's story

Ever since he retired from the Marines after 30 years of service and several tours of duty, Claude has doted on his garden. His wife loves it because it keeps her busy canning and they are never at a loss for vegetables. His neighbors love it because it's not unusual for them to wake up on Saturday morning and find grocery bags full of tomatoes, cucumbers, squash and corn sitting on their front porches.

One word to describe Claude would have to be "physical." He stayed in great shape while in the Marines, always passing his physical exams with flying colors. Even at age 59, Claude spends mornings walking through his garden, weeding, picking or planting. He rests in the afternoons with a good book. Then, in the early evening, he and his wife often take a long walk. He also goes to his doctor for regular checkups. His only problems seem to be slightly elevated blood pressure and cholesterol levels. His constant good health was one reason it took Claude so long to take his slight chest pain seriously.

What is heart disease?

Heart disease is the leading killer of Americans. Although heart-related deaths have decreased in the last 15 years, heart disease still kills nearly as many Americans as all other diseases combined. Even though you may think you are in good health, like Claude, you may be at risk for heart disease without even knowing it.

As you read this page, your heart is pumping blood throughout your body approximately 80 times per minute—that's over 115,000 times in one day or more than 30 million times each year. To prevent heart disease, it's important to take precautions every day, whether you're healthy or not. (See Chapter Two for more information about this.) Because it's a large muscle, your heart needs lots of nourishment to keep up its pace. Anything you put into your body that clogs your coronary arteries (straw-sized vessels on the surface of and within the heart muscle) can make your heart's job more difficult, eventually causing health problems. When something goes wrong that blocks or decreases the amount of blood, which provides nourishment to the heart itself, problems can occur.

Your heart is a strong muscle that lies behind your breastbone in the left center of your chest. It serves as a pump with four rooms or chambers, two on top and two on the bottom. Each upper chamber is known as an atrium, the lower chambers as ventricles. Your upper chambers receive blood from your veins and serve as reservoirs. The lower chambers, ventricles, are the pumping chambers of your heart. Your left ventricle pumps oxygenated blood to all the parts of your body, except your lungs. Your right ventricle pumps blood coming from your body to your lungs so that your blood can be oxygenated. The two ventricles are separated by a wall of muscle about half an inch thick, called the septum.

Your blood goes from one chamber to another and out of your heart through four valves, which act like one-way doors, letting blood flow through them in only one direction. Each valve has two or three flaps, the cusps, which open and close with the force of the blood in your heart. The two valves between your atria and ventricles are called the mitral valve and the tricuspid valve. The aortic valve opens to let blood flow out of your left ventricle and into your aorta (the main vessel supplying blood to your body). The valve that allows blood to flow out of your right ventricle to your lungs is called the pulmonary artery (the main blood vessel supplying blood to your lungs).

In general, there are four things that can go wrong with your heart:

1. Your coronary arteries (blood vessels supplying the heart) can get clogged.
2. Your heart muscle itself can get too big and weaken.
3. The valves within your heart can get stuck or not open properly.

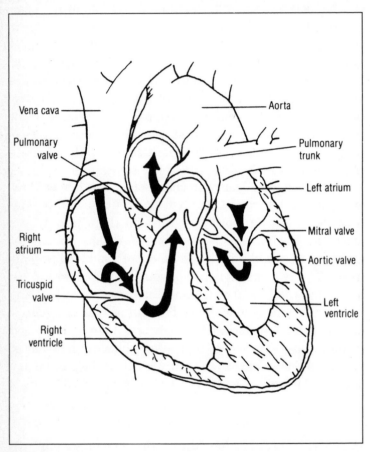

FIGURE 4A

The heart.
Reprinted with permission of the American Heart Association.

4. You can develop a disorder of the electrical impulses of your heart, which can result in irregular heart rhythms.

Claude listens to reason

The first time the pain occurred, Claude was tilling his garden, preparing it for winter. The pain started in his chest and radiated out in a slow burn toward his arms and jaw. Experiencing difficulty in breathing, Claude immediately shut down the tiller and sat down in the shade. Within ten to fifteen minutes, he felt better. He put away the tiller and finished the job later in the week. The next time the pain came, he was carrying bags of fertilizer to the shed. Again, Claude stopped the activity, rested awhile and soon felt better. The third time occurred during one of his evening walks with his wife. She was concerned and asked him to make an appointment to see his doctor. By this time, Claude was concerned enough to agree.

When Claude described his attacks of pain, his doctor had a good idea what was wrong, but to be sure, he ordered a battery of tests. Sure enough, Claude had been experiencing angina attacks, which occur because of a lack of blood flowing to nourish the heart muscle. The doctor explained to Claude that a combination of his age and high blood pressure had contributed to the condition. He prescribed nitroglycerin tablets to be taken when the pain occurred.

Today, Claude carries nitroglycerin tablets with him wherever he goes and takes them only when necessary. He eats foods with low or no cholesterol or fat, and he continues to work in his garden as much as ever. He's even tilled up more of the backyard in order to make room for five more rows—his grandchildren want to plant pumpkins and watermelon to sell roadside for extra money.

Black men are at greater risk of death from heart disease

According to the American Heart Association, there were 930,477 deaths from cardiovascular disease in 1990. Heart disease costs the country approximately $43 billion each year in direct and indirect costs. "Coronary heart disease death rates are higher among men than among women and are higher among blacks than among whites," according to *Healthy People 2000: National Health Promotion and Disease Prevention Objectives* (the nation's health strategy, published in 1990). "In 1987, the age-adjusted coronary heart disease death rate for black men was 208 per 100,000, compared to 185 per 100,000 for white men. (An age standardization method is used to validate statistical comparison among rates by assuming the same age distribution occurs in the different groups compared.) The death rate for black women was 129 per 100,000 compared to 90 per 100,000 for white women."[1]

The nation's health strategy also says that "while the coronary heart disease death rate has declined steadily over the past 20 years for white men, the decline has slowed substantially over the past 10 years for black men, black women and white women."[2]

Because these declines in deaths related to heart disease are primarily due to lifestyle changes, the differences between black and white men may be due to the fact that in recent years, white men have been assumed, both by the media and the medical community, to be at greatest risk for the disease. As a result, white men may be targeted more for treatment and prevention than women and blacks. However, as you can tell from the above statistics, black men are at even greater risk of heart-related deaths than white men.

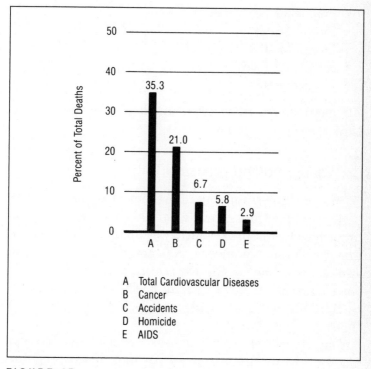

FIGURE 4B

Leading causes of death for black males in 1988.
1993 Heart and Stroke Facts and Statistics, copyright © 1992 American Heart Association. Reprinted with permission.

How can I prevent heart disease?

Because making lifestyle changes can greatly reduce your risk of death from heart disease, it's important to know how you can make these changes a part of your life. In the second section of this chapter, we will discuss stroke, another form of cardiovascular disease. Following are simple prevention techniques you can use to prevent both of these disorders:

- ◆ Stop smoking
- ◆ Fight obesity
- ◆ Lower "bad" cholesterol
- ◆ Avoid fast food
- ◆ Reduce your stress

For more information about all these prevention techniques, see Chapter Two.

Control high blood pressure

Another important way to prevent heart disease is to keep your blood pressure at a normal level. Hypertension (high blood pressure), which we discussed in depth in Chapter Three, is a major risk factor of heart disease and stroke, according to *The Report of the Secretary's Task Force on Black & Minority Health*. The prevalence of hypertension among adult blacks aged 18–74 years is 1.4 times greater than among whites.

Your chance of having a heart attack rises as your blood pressure rises. If you have high blood pressure, you have a three to four times greater risk of developing coronary heart disease than someone with a normal blood pressure. Being hypertensive also makes you seven times more likely to have a stroke. There are several strategies you can use to lower your blood pressure. See Chapter Three for a more comprehensive discussion of these.

What about unavoidable risks?

In addition to risk factors that can be reduced or eliminated from your life, there are others that cannot be changed or are difficult to change, such as socioeconomic class, heredity, age and being male. Blacks who have lower educational levels and low incomes usually have higher blood pressure. Living in areas of instability and high social stress, as well as constantly grappling with educational and occupational insecurity, may increase your blood pressure, making you at greater risk for heart disease and stroke. If you're in a low socioeconomic class, you may also not have access to quality medical care. Blacks are reported to make fewer visits to their doctors, and many regard medical care as inaccessible.

Unfortunately, if heart disease runs in your family, you may have an increased risk of heart disease. It is also important to remember that heart disease is diagnosed more often in people over age 50. Although you can't control your age, you can be sure to see a physician regularly. Even if some of your personal risk factors cannot be changed, it's important to be aware of the controllable risk factors we've mentioned here. You can decrease your likelihood of developing heart disease and increase your likelihood of living a long, healthy life.

How do I know if I have heart disease?

One way to tell if you have a particular illness or disease is to look for signs (something visibly *noticed*) and symptoms (changes in the way you *feel*). With heart disease, this can be confusing because many times, symptoms of other health disorders mimic those associated with heart disease. The primary indications of heart disease are:

1. Rapid pounding of your heart
2. Swelling in your legs
3. Shortness of breath
4. Pain located generally in the center of your chest
5. Fainting

If you are experiencing any of these, this does not automatically mean you have heart disease. Only by working with your physician or primary health care provider will you be able to determine exactly what caused the physical changes you are experiencing. Heart disease is not something to be taken lightly. If you have experienced any of the sensations listed above, seek counsel from a medical professional immediately.

Medical detection techniques

There are many different ways your health care professional can determine if you have heart disease. The first, least expensive method is simply listening to your heart. Your heart makes two sounds—"lubb" and "dubb." These sounds are made by the closing of the four valves we mentioned earlier. If your doctor hears sounds other than these through the stethoscope, it may indicate that you have a heart problem.

If your doctor suspects heart trouble, there are many other tests he or she can order to make an accurate diagnosis. A few of the more common ones follow.

1. An *electrocardiogram (EKG or ECG)* records your heart's electrical activity to help your doctor detect any changes in the pattern of your heart's rhythm. When giving you an EKG, your medical professional will attach small wires to various areas of your body. These wires will be attached to the electrocardiogram machine, which will trace the patterns of electrical activity within your heart.

2. *Chest X rays* can show if your heart is enlarged or displaced within your chest cavity.

3. Your doctor can also order a test called an *echocardiogram,* which, by using sound waves, can detect motion of your heart and details of its valves and wall.

4. Your doctor may also ask you to undergo a *cardiac catheterization,* a procedure in which dye is injected into your heart and its vessels. X rays taken while the dye is in your body can portray your heart and its vessels in detail.

If, after the test results come back from one of these procedures, you are diagnosed with heart disease, it's important to make lifestyle changes and comply closely with the treatment plan your doctor prescribes. Otherwise, the consequences can be deadly.

Malcolm's story

The day of Malcolm's company picnic was glorious. The lakesite had horseshoes, a pool, badminton and volleyball for all the employees and their families.

From the volleyball court, Malcolm looked over at his wife and smiled. Then he noticed a slightly overweight man sitting at the picnic table next to her. The man's hand was resting over his chest and his skin was very pale. More importantly, there was panic in the man's eyes. Malcolm had seen these very same signs in his own father when he was having a heart attack.

Malcolm took off running toward the man. Over his shoulder, he yelled to his surprised teammates to call an ambulance, although he knew that, by the time the paramedics arrived, it could be too late. He yelled to his wife, who turned immediately toward the man, who was already slumping off the picnic table bench. She caught him just in time to keep his head from bumping the concrete patio. Malcolm reached the man and immediately searched for his pulse. There wasn't one. He stretched the man out on the ground, tore open his shirt, loosened the man's belt, and began CPR, which he had been trained in at his former job. Since no one else at the picnic knew CPR, Malcolm used the one-person CPR method of two breaths for every fifteen compressions on the man's chest. He kept administering CPR until he heard sirens in the distance. The color was coming back to the man's face. Malcolm stopped and checked for a pulse. The man's pulse, although weak, had returned.

Soon after, paramedics arrived and transported the man to the hospital. It turned out the man, whose name was Larry, worked on the floor below Malcolm's office. Larry survived the trip to the hospital and recovered nicely. Today, Larry has changed his diet, lost some weight and is exercising regularly. After that weekend, Malcolm's office sponsored a mandatory CPR class for all its employees.

Saving lives with CPR

Sometimes, the heart completely stops beating or simply quivers, which means that although there is movement from the heart, it is not pumping blood. When the heart stops, cardiopulmonary resuscitation (CPR) can maintain blood flow to the rest of the body until medical therapy is instituted.

Getting medical help quickly is very important when the heart stops. Even though a health care facility may be nearby, there may not be enough time to get professional help. For such an occasion, CPR is more than a valuable thing to know—it is essential for life. You can never be sure when someone's heart may stop beating and CPR will be necessary. It takes four to six minutes for the brain to suffer irreversible damage. Brain death or a persistent vegetative state could occur if the victim does not receive medical treatment within 10 minutes. Heart muscle tissue can die within five minutes after the heart stops beating. Unfortunately, CPR is helpful only when someone who knows CPR is present and ready for action when the victim collapses.

Your cells need oxygen to survive. If someone's heart stops beating, it is necessary to apply CPR to keep the heart pumping blood to the lungs and brain until medical therapy can be instituted to start the heart beating on its own again. Consider taking a CPR course, such as those offered by the American Red Cross, for hands-on experience—you could quite possibly save someone's life. Also, suggest to your employer or employees the possibility of having a CPR instructor come to your office to teach you and your coworkers this lifesaving skill.

Types of heart disease

There are different causes and types of heart diseases. Some, called congenital heart defects, are unavoidable and caused by heart defects at birth. Congenital heart defects can be genetic or developmental. Research is currently being done to diagnose and treat these disorders in children before they are even born. Other types of heart disease are caused by lifestyle factors, which we've already reviewed. If you have been diagnosed with heart disease, there are many conditions you may have.

Atherosclerosis

Atherosclerosis occurs when the inner lining of your arteries is injured as a result of high blood pressure, elevated cholesterol or toxins from smoke inhalation. Scarring can occur, especially from smoking, and cholesterol deposits can cause your arteries to stiffen and their inner walls to narrow or clog. If your artery walls have narrowed, your blood may clot in its attempt to pass through the artery. This can partially or completely obstruct the vessel, which can cause a heart attack or stroke.

When atherosclerosis blocks one of your coronary arteries (vessels located on the surface of and in your heart, which supply your heart with nourishment), part of your heart's blood supply can be cut off. This can produce a symptom called angina or a heart attack (see below).

Angina

Angina, from the Greek root *anchonē*, means strangulation. Angina is a sensation—a heaviness or tightness—in your chest, usually felt over your breastbone or next

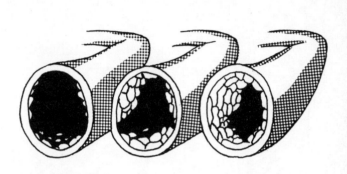

In atherosclerosis, plaque builds up in arteries over time and may partially or totally block blood flow.

FIGURE 4C

Atherosclerosis.
1993 Heart and Stroke Facts and Statistics, copyright © 1992 American Heart Association. Reprinted with permission.

to your breastbone, sometimes radiating down the left arm and shoulder or spreading in fan fashion to your jaw. Angina is experienced differently by different people. It is generally described, however, as a frightening and oppressive feeling that can be accompanied by sweating, aching and shortness of breath. It has also been described as a "full" feeling.

Since angina attacks occur when your heart muscle doesn't receive as much blood as it needs, functions that require more blood flow, such as exercise, anxiety or eating, are most likely to bring on an attack. Angina can also occur while you are resting or sleeping, and may be a warning sign of a pending heart attack.

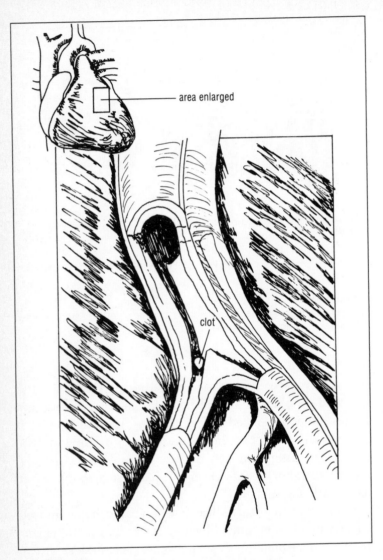

area enlarged

clot

FIGURE 4D

A coronary artery that has become narrowed or clogged.
"Heart Attack," copyright © 1992 American Heart Association. Reprinted
with permission.

Heart attack

When atherosclerosis (above) becomes so severe that it closes off one of your coronary arteries, a heart attack occurs. Also called a myocardial infarction, a heart attack sometimes produces symptoms that are similar to angina, but worse. The part of your heart that is served by the blocked artery is now cut off from its blood supply. While damage to your heart muscle can begin in only a few minutes, we know that this damage can be reversed within the first six hours, by using a class of drugs called "clot busters."

One of the major symptoms of a heart attack is pain; however, the pain can be severe, mild, so slight that it is dismissed as indigestion or an aching muscle, or even absent. Sometimes, instead of pain, a heart attack victim may complain of chest discomfort or tightness. But you don't have to experience pain or symptoms to suffer a heart attack. One out of every four heart attack victims experiences no symptoms at all. These heart attacks are called "silent." One difference between angina and a heart attack is that the pain from a heart attack will usually not lessen when you take a nitroglycerin tablet or rest.

Massive heart attack victims describe the experience as a very heavy, crushing feeling; the pain, they say, is usually centered under their breastbone. Some heart attack victims report pain in their back, between their shoulders, as well as in their left arm, jaw, shoulder and in back of their neck. Heart attack victims may also experience sweating, shortness of breath, nausea and vomiting.

Speed in medical assistance is essential when treating a heart attack. If you think that you or someone you know has experienced a heart attack, don't wait around to see if the condition eases or if the symptoms return. Seek medical attention immediately because the heart may stop or beat so irregularly that the brain won't receive any blood for nourishment. While you are waiting for assistance to arrive, calm the victim as much as possible.

Heart failure

Heart failure occurs when your heart fails to perform adequately as a pump. This can result in the backup of fluid in your lungs, causing shortness of breath or swelling in your legs or abdomen. Heart failure can be caused by inadequate blood flow to the heart muscle itself, permanent scars, or inflammation (destruction caused by infection or other problems), which all lead to an unhealthy heart muscle. Heart failure can result from prolonged high blood pressure, coronary artery disease, a viral illness, alcohol overuse, other toxins or congenital heart disease.

Not all people who experience heart failure die from the condition. It only means that the pumping action of their heart is not adequate and needs to be treated.

Enlargement of the heart

Retired Supreme Court Justice Thurgood Marshall—the first black Supreme Court Justice, appointed by President Lyndon B. Johnson in 1967—died in 1993 of heart failure due to an enlarged heart. He was 84 years old.

A major cause of heart enlargement is overwork. Just as weightlifting causes your muscles to become bigger and stronger, when your heart has to work harder to pump blood through your body (when you have hypertension, for example), the muscle builds and your heart becomes bigger. Unfortunately, in the case of the heart, bigger is not better. The bigger your heart grows, the more difficult it is for it to work efficiently. In fact, if your heart is enlarged, that means it is weakened and may be less able to perform its functions. (To gain a better understanding of how to avoid or lessen the effects of high blood pressure, see Chapter Three.)

Arrhythmia

An arrhythmia is an abnormal heartbeat. A normal heartbeat begins in your right atrium. Special pacemaker cells then send out an electrical signal. This signal causes your heart to contract. Each contraction is one heartbeat. The "lubb-dubb" sound you hear when you listen through a stethoscope is caused by your atria contracting a split second before your ventricles do. This fractional time difference allows the doors or valves of your atria to slam shut before the valves of your ventricles open.

An arrhythmia occurs when there is any variation to this "lubb-dubb" rhythm. Sometimes arrhythmias are dangerous because they can cause your heart to pump less efficiently. They are often associated with symptoms such as dizziness, passing out or chest pain. *Ventricular fibrillation,* the most serious type of rhythm disorder, can cause your ventricles to quiver and prevent your heart from pumping out any blood at all. When a patient has ventricular fibrillation, it may be necessary to "jumpstart" his or her heart with CPR or an electric shock.

An artificial pacemaker is another possible treatment

for arrhythmia. A pacemaker is a tiny device that is placed near your heart. Some types of pacemakers stimulate the heart continuously, while others work only if the heart rate falls below a certain level.

Heart valve disorders

Your valves, or the doors located within your heart, are also potential danger zones. Congenital heart diseases (heart defects present at birth) and rheumatic heart disease can cause your valves to get stuck, or to fail to open and close correctly. Many congenital diseases, such as a hole in your heart, can be corrected with surgery. Other heart valve disorders that at one time commonly resulted from strep infections, such as rheumatic fever, have been largely eliminated in the United States since the introduction of penicillin. However, these disorders are still common in underdeveloped countries with poor access to health care.

SECTION TWO:
STROKE

Stroke

Stroke is another form of cardiovascular disease. A stroke occurs when your brain's blood supply is interrupted by a blocked blood vessel or when a blood vessel in your brain bursts, causing hemorrhage. When these things happen, your brain cells are deprived of oxygen and they die.

According to the National Stroke Association, stroke is the third leading cause of death by disease in the

United States and the number-one cause of adult disability. Between 500,000 and 600,000 people in the United States have a stroke every year. Approximately one-third of stroke victims die within a month after the attack, while the remaining two-thirds of stroke victims are likely to suffer some type of disability.

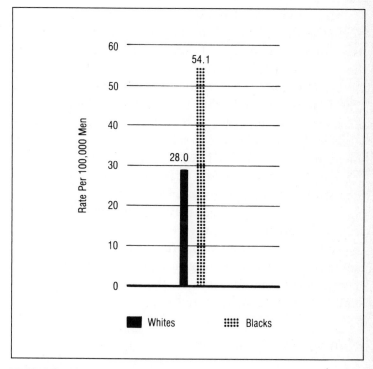

FIGURE 4E

Age-adjusted stroke death rates.
1993 Heart and Stroke Facts and Statistics, copyright © 1992 American Heart Association. Reprinted with permission.

What is my chance of having a stroke?

Your risk of having a stroke is greater if you are black, male, over 65 years of age, have diabetes, or if you or someone in your family has already had a stroke. These risk factors are things you cannot change.

Also, if you live in an area called the "Stroke Belt"— a region that includes twelve southeastern states—you are more likely to have a stroke. The "Stroke Belt" includes certain areas in Alabama, Arkansas, Florida, Georgia, Indiana, Kentucky, Louisiana, Mississippi, North Carolina, South Carolina, Tennessee and Virginia. According to the National Stroke Association, blacks in the "Stroke Belt" are two times more likely to have strokes and more likely to die from strokes than whites. This is most probably due to the diet of blacks within these areas, which tends to be extremely high in cholesterols and saturated fats. Stroke rates among blacks are the highest in the United States. This is according to the Office of Minority Health (OMH), which has a task force that studies the disparity between the health status of blacks and other Americans. Black men are also almost twice as likely to die from strokes as white men. As mentioned before, this may be because of a variety of factors, including lifestyle, diet, poor access to medical care, lack of awareness and research in the area of black men's health, and racial discrimination.

Warning signs of a stroke

There are many signs and symptoms of an impending stroke. The American Heart Association reports that you can possibly avert or lessen the damage from a stroke by recognizing the following warning signals and getting immediate medical attention:

1. Sudden blurred or decreased vision in one or both eyes
2. Numbness, weakness and paralysis of the face, upper or lower limbs, on one or both sides of the body
3. Difficulty speaking or understanding
4. Dizziness, loss of balance or an unexplained fall
5. Difficulty swallowing
6. Headache (usually severe and of abrupt onset) or an unexplained change in the pattern of headaches[3]

If you experience any of these symptoms, alone or in any combination, consult your doctor immediately.

Types of strokes

There are many different types of strokes.

1. *Cerebral thrombosis* is the most common type of stroke. Thrombotic strokes account for 60 percent of all strokes and generally occur in people over the age of 65. A thrombotic stroke occurs when an artery leading to your brain is blocked or clogged by a blood clot, or when the wall of one of your arteries thickens. (For more information about this phenomenon, see the section on atherosclerosis earlier in this chapter.) This type of stroke generally occurs during the morning or at night, when your blood pressure is at its lowest.
2. A *cerebral embolism* may occur when an artery leading to your brain is clogged by an embolus, which is a blood clot that has traveled from another area of your body.
3. *Cerebral hemorrhages* occur less frequently than the

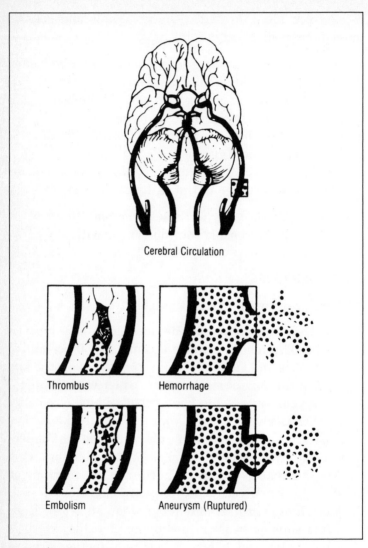

Cerebral Circulation

Thrombus

Hemorrhage

Embolism

Aneurysm (Ruptured)

FIGURE 4F

Different kinds of stroke.
1993 Heart and Stroke Facts and Statistics, copyright © 1992 American Heart Association. Reprinted with permission.

two stroke forms listed above. A cerebral hemorrhage is usually the result of an artery bursting in your brain. This type of stroke is caused by an aneurysm, a weak spot in the wall of an artery that balloons out. Aneurysms may develop over a period of years and are often caused by high blood pressure, which can stretch out weak spots in your blood vessels.

When the artery bursts, the area the artery leads to is deprived of blood. If the artery leads to the brain, it can cause brain cells to die. Since your brain often cannot repair itself when deprived of oxygen, there is a chance that a victim of cerebral hemorrhage will suffer brain damage or death. Another complication of cerebral hemorrhage is that excess blood from the broken vessel may accumulate and cause pressure on the brain.

Treatment for heart disease and stroke

There are many options available when it comes to treating heart disease and stroke. What your doctor prescribes will depend on your specific problem. Treatments include changes in diet, exercise, medication, special procedures, rehabilitation and surgery. Recent advances in medical research have provided many unique opportunities to cure and control cardiovascular diseases.

Conclusion

If you have heart disease or a stroke, it does not mean your life is over. As with Claude, the quality of your life will depend on whether or not you are willing to take an active role in your health care. Monitor your blood pressure, control your blood cholesterol through diet and exercise, eat healthy foods and don't smoke. Even if your doctor says that you're perfectly healthy, you still need to live a healthy lifestyle to prevent heart disease from striking sometime in the future.

If you fall into one or more of the risk groups for heart disease or stroke, pay close attention to the preventive measures we've discussed here and in Chapter Two. Follow the advice of your doctor, health educator or specialist. By working together, you will increase your chance of preventing and treating cardiovascular disease.

Resources

American College of Cardiology
9111 Old Georgetown Rd.
Bethesda, MD 20814-1699
(800) 253-4636
(301) 897-5400

American Heart Association
7320 Greenville Ave.
Dallas, TX 75231-4599
(214) 373-6300
(800) 242-8721

(The Association offers information, referrals, booklets, brochures and community education programs.)

The Mended Hearts, Inc.
7320 Greenville Ave.
Dallas, TX 75231

(This is a support group for people who have gone through a heart attack, heart surgery or angioplasty.

Look up the chapter near you or write to the organization for more information.)

>National Health Information Center
>8455 Colesville Road, Suite 935
>Silver Spring, MD 20910

(Write to the Center for free health information.)

>National Heart, Lung and Blood Institute
>Information Center
>PO Box 30105
>Bethesda, MD 20824-0105
>(301) 251-1222

(The Information Center provides free information and materials about cardiovascular disease and associated risk factors.)

>National Institute of Neurological Disorders and
>   Stroke
>Office of Scientific and Health Reports
>PO Box 5801
>Bethesda, MD 20824
>(800) 352-9424
>(301) 496-5751

(The Institute offers free brochures about strokes.)

>National Rehabilitation Information Center
>8455 Colesville Rd., Suite 935
>Silver Spring, MD 20910
>(800) 34-NARIC voice/TDD
>(301) 588-9284

(The Center provides some brochures, but mainly provides article reprints, for a fee.)

National Stroke Association
8480 East Orchard Road, Suite 1000
Englewood, CO 80111-5015
(800) 787-6537
(303) 771-1700

(This Association offers free screenings in hospitals, stroke support groups, videos, pamphlets, booklets and brochures.)

5

Diabetes

Jack, a diabetic in control

"He was tall, big and dashing and I loved him so much," said Deborah, sharing memories of her godfather. "I was a teenager when I heard he had diabetes and I didn't understand. I'd never heard him talk about his disease, and he never seemed sick to me. I thought my parents were talking about someone else when they said Jack had diabetes."

What is diabetes?

Unless you are diabetic, you probably can't explain the disease. It's not something you can see. Most people only know that it has something to do with insulin and sugar. Many people still believe that diabetes is not serious.

Maybe you've heard people say, "He'll be okay in a few minutes. He's just got 'sugar problems.' Give him some candy." Well, that's not all there is to it.

When you are diagnosed with diabetes, it means that something is wrong with the way your body secretes insulin. Insulin is a chemical (hormone) normally produced by your pancreas to control your blood sugar level. If you have diabetes, your body may have a shortage or a complete lack of insulin. Or, the insulin you do have may not be capable of doing its job properly. When you eat, your body breaks food into glucose, a type of sugar that enters your bloodstream as an energy source. If your body lacks insulin, the level of this sugar builds up steadily, with no way of balancing out naturally.

Diabetes and blacks

As of 1992, approximately one out of every 20 Americans (totaling 13 million people) had diabetes. Diabetes was also the sixth leading underlying cause of death in the United States, leading to approximately 37,000 fatalities.[1] Many steps have been taken to control and prevent diabetes, but there is still no cure.

Diabetes affects American minorities (African-Americans, Hispanics and Native Americans) more than it does whites. Although diabetes is the sixth leading cause of death in the United States overall, in the black community it ranks third. (Cardiovascular disease and cancer are the first and second leading killers of blacks, respectively.)

Diabetes-related deaths among black Americans were 65 per 100,000 in 1986. The prevalence of the disease is 35 percent higher in the black population than among whites, according to the Secretary's Task Force on Black and Minority Health.[2] One reason diabetes is such a significant health problem is that it is a major risk factor for other life-threatening diseases, such as atherosclerosis (heart and blood vessel disease) and hypertension (high blood pressure). See Chapter Three and Chapter Four for more information about these illnesses.

A diabetes patient faces not only the threat of a shortened life, but also the increased chance of developing additional medical complications. Several studies report that diabetes-related complications are more frequent among blacks. These complications include blindness, gangrene requiring amputations, and chronic renal (kidney) failure.

In 1987 diabetes accounted for approximately 10,000 new cases of kidney disease in the United States and 30 percent of end stage renal disease (ESRD) or kidney failure cases. The incidence of ESRD caused by diabetes has increased about 10 percent each year since 1983.[3] (For more information about kidney disease, see Chapter Eight.)

What causes diabetes and how can I prevent it?

No one knows exactly what causes diabetes, though certain people have a greater tendency to get the disease than others. Heredity is a major causal factor. Other contributing factors to diabetes include rapid weight gain, inflammation of the pancreas, or other illnesses. In these cases, following the guidelines for general good health outlined in Chapter Two may help you to prevent or delay the onset of the disease. Also, constantly keeping your weight at a healthy level and staying away from "quick cure" diets may help to prevent the disease. Eight out of ten people who are diagnosed with adult onset diabetes are overweight. Following the guidelines in Chapter Two may also help you prevent other illnesses that can lead to diabetes.

What we do know for sure is that diabetes is not communicable. You can't catch it, and you can't give it to anyone else. If you are not diabetic, you can still be close to someone who is like Jack, without any risk to yourself.

Types of diabetes

There are two main types of diabetes: Type I and Type II. There are also a few secondary types of diabetes.

Type I diabetes

Type I diabetes, also known as insulin-dependent diabetes, usually occurs in children and young adults, although it can strike at any age. Approximately one million people in the United States have this type of diabetes.

If you are a Type I (insulin-dependent) diabetic, you have little or no insulin in your body and must take daily insulin injections to survive. When insulin is not available, the cells in your body can virtually starve (because sugar isn't allowed to pass into the cells) while your liver produces excess amounts of glucose, which remains useless in your blood.

How do I know if I have Type I diabetes?

According to the American Diabetes Association, these are the common symptoms of a Type I diabetic:

- frequent urination (and/or bed-wetting in children)
- extreme hunger
- extreme thirst
- extreme weight loss
- weakness and fatigue
- feeling edgy and having mood changes
- feeling sick to your stomach and vomiting
- blurred vision

If you experience any of these symptoms, see your doctor immediately.

Type II diabetes

Type II, or non-insulin-dependent diabetes, is the most common type of the disease and occurs in more than 90 percent of all known diabetics. Type II diabetes usually occurs in overweight adults older than age 40, which is why it's sometimes referred to as "adult onset diabetes." The majority of blacks who have diabetes have Type II diabetes.

Type II diabetes occurs when your pancreas does not make enough insulin or when your body can't adequately use the insulin your pancreas does produce. If you have Type II diabetes, however, your condition may be managed through your diet. The quality and length of your life will depend primarily on how committed you are to being an active participant in your own health care. By taking control, many Type II diabetics have lived full, happy, healthy lives, often living longer than their friends who don't have the disease. By following the diet and lifestyle recommended to keep your disorder in check, you will benefit your overall health as well.

Obesity is a major cause of Type II diabetes. In fact,

more than 80 percent of all people with Type II diabetes are obese. Keeping your weight down may be a key factor in preventing the disease because insulin does not function properly if you're overweight. On the outside of each of your cells are areas called insulin receptor sites. As you might imagine, these sites are where insulin attaches itself to each cell and allows the blood glucose to enter. If you are obese, these insulin receptor sites are less effective because your body's ability to transport glucose into the cell is diminished. Therefore, your body may become resistant to insulin. (See Chapter Two for more information about weight reduction.)

How do I know if I have Type II diabetes?

In some families, Type II diabetes is hereditary, and several members of each generation may develop the disease. If your family has a history of diabetes, you should be tested periodically, especially after you reach age 40, or if you're overweight. Unlike with Type I, the symptoms in Type II diabetes are sometimes so mild that you don't realize you're sick. If you are at risk for diabetes, look for the following signs (a physical change visibly noticed) and symptoms (changes in the way you feel) of Type II diabetes, as noted by the U.S. Department of Health and Human Services and the American Diabetes Association:

◆ fatigue
◆ frequent urination, especially at night
◆ unusual thirst
◆ sudden weight loss
◆ blurred vision or any change in sight

◆ slow healing of infections of the skin, gums and urinary tract
◆ tingling or numbness in feet, legs or fingers
◆ frequent skin infections
◆ irritability

If you detect any of these symptoms, see your doctor immediately.

Sometimes, however, you can be diabetic without experiencing any noticeable changes in your health. For instance, you may not notice any symptoms, but you may have a medical history of glucose (sugar) in your urine, or a gradual increase in your blood glucose level over several months or years. In older patients, a doctor may discover diabetes during a routine physical exam, or when the patient is in the hospital for another reason. In these cases, you may have experienced only slight fatigue, or frequent thirst and urination. Or, perhaps you did not experience any symptoms at all. These cases are common—which is yet another reason why it's important to be tested for diabetes on a regular basis.

How to control diabetes

Diabetes is serious, but it is not a death sentence. If you are diabetic, your health is very dependent on how you choose to manage your condition. You are in control. You can sit back and let the disease run its course—and ruin your life as well—or you can pay close attention to what your body needs and take care of it.

One way of looking at your "life with diabetes" is that it's the kind of lifestyle everyone should adopt. If you're diabetic, it's essential that you eat well, exercise regularly and pay close attention to the signs and signals of your body in order to effectively manage your health. Having diabetes can be a great excuse to get your whole family involved in living a healthy lifestyle.

If you have diabetes, you're part of a team that includes your physician, health educator, nutritionist, eye doctor, foot doctor and others who specialize in common complications of diabetes. There will be times in your life that you need the help of all your teammates, but you are the team captain. Before seeking help, you'll need to first understand your condition. You're the one who needs to monitor your body day in and day out, and become aware of the warning signs that signal that it's time to rely on someone else from the team.

Monitoring your condition

To effectively monitor your health, begin making routine visits to your doctor three or four times a year. If you develop additional health problems, you may need to visit your doctor more often. Your doctor will usually check your weight, blood pressure and pulse and listen to your heart at every visit. He or she will also examine your eyes and feet. (We'll explain why later in this chapter.)

One of your jobs as team captain will be to monitor your blood glucose (HGM—Home Glucose Monitoring) two or three times a week, perhaps more often, if you're taking insulin. Your health care professional (doctor, nurse, diabetes educator, etc.) will counsel you about how often you need to test your blood sugar. Every diabetes patient should have an established schedule geared to his or her individual needs.

How do I test my blood sugar?

There are numerous products available that you can use to test your blood glucose levels. These include lancets and holders, which you use to prick your finger to get a small drop of blood; test strips, which you read by comparing the color on the strip to a color chart; and blood glucose monitors, which automatically read test strips and show your exact blood glucose level. Your health care professional can help you determine the method that is best for you and instruct you how to use it.

Most doctors agree that blood glucose testing is the best and most accurate method to control your blood glucose levels. Maintain a record for yourself, as well as one to show your doctor when you go for a checkup. This data will be helpful in planning your personal health program.

Once a year, you should get a thorough physical examination. Your doctor should pay special attention to your cholesterol and triglyceride levels. Ideally, your cholesterol level should be below 200 milligrams and your triglyceride level below 150 milligrams. You can also have an EKG (electrocardiogram) and other diagnostic tests done to evaluate your risk of any long-term complications.

You should have the health of your kidneys checked with urine and blood tests. Also, your physician should do an in-depth evaluation of your blood pressure several different times. If your blood pressure is above 130/85, he or she will usually put you on a program to reduce it to a lower, "normal" blood pressure level.

You should also have your eyes thoroughly examined once a year by an eye doctor (ophthalmologist). This is very important, since treatments are available that can help prevent blindness, a common complication of diabetes.

The importance of insulin

Insulin is a hormone that helps your body use glucose (sugar) for energy and keeps your blood sugar at a healthy level. Your pancreas produces insulin, then sends it into your bloodstream when needed. As the amount of sugar in your blood rises, your pancreas detects this and sends out a "message" via insulin into your bloodstream. This insulin "message" causes all your cells to take the sugar out of your blood and use it for energy. When the level of sugar in your blood is low, your pancreas does not send insulin so your body preserves the little sugar you have instead of using it for energy. You always have some sugar in your bloodstream. Your brain cannot function without blood sugar.

When you develop diabetes, either your pancreas becomes unable to produce insulin, or your cells are unable to receive the insulin "message." As a result, your body can no longer use the food you eat correctly and you cannot control the amount of sugar in your bloodstream. This defect can affect many other parts of your body.

How do I know if I need insulin injections?

If you are a Type I diabetic, you are insulin-dependent. This means you will need a daily injection of insulin. Some Type II diabetics also need to take insulin. Most insulin taken by diabetics is human insulin, made by recombinant DNA. If you are taking insulin therapy, your doctor will develop a custom-made plan to best suit your needs. Through blood sugar tests, you and your doctor will be able to tell how much insulin you will need throughout each day.

In managing your diabetes, it is essential for you to monitor your own blood glucose level (SMBG). The results of SMBG tests can be used to pinpoint problems in your health care methods. Once you've identified any existing problems in your therapy, you and your doctor can work to correct them by making changes in your diet, exercise, other areas of your lifestyle or your insulin dose.

Jack takes diabetes in stride

When Deborah saw her godfather again, after learning about his condition, she asked him about his diabetes. Jack said he'd had it since he was a teenager. "It's nothing for you to worry about. It takes me less time to take care of my condition than it takes you to put on your makeup," he assured her. Indeed, Deborah could never remember having seen her godfather devote any time at all to his condition. In fact, Jack was probably the most energetic, happy-go-lucky man she had ever met.

Curious, Deborah asked Jack to show her how he treated his condition. He was delighted with her interest. He had already taken his insulin shot that morning, so he agreed to call her when he took his next injection.

When the time came, he showed her the insulin supply he kept in the refrigerator and the individually wrapped syringes stored in the medicine cabinet. Jack pulled up his shirt and scrubbed an area on his abdomen with soap and water. Deborah, wary of needles, flinched when Jack pushed the needle into his abdomen, but Jack never reacted. "I've been doing this for years," said Jack. "It's like brushing my teeth."

How do I take insulin injections?

Your doctor or nurse will show you how to take insulin injections. You will need to inject your insulin into the fatty tissue under your skin, instead of into a vein. By doing this, you allow for better, more even absorption of the insulin into your bloodstream. Make sure you clean the top of the bottle of insulin and the area of skin where you will be injecting yourself with rubbing alcohol, or soap and water. Each time you take insulin, change the place you inject yourself. If you use the same site each time, your skin can get irritated. The abdomen is the area where most diabetics prefer to inject themselves, because absorpion is slower there than areas such as your arm, leg or hip. When insulin is absorbed into your body quickly, its effects will not last as long.

Here's how

To take an insulin injection, follow these simple steps:

1. Pull back on the plunger of the needle to the number of units you need.
2. Push the needle into the bottle and depress the plunger, which pushes air into the bottle.
3. Turn the insulin bottle upside down and draw the required amount of insulin into the syringe.
4. Tap the syringe, still inside the bottle, which will send the air bubbles to the top.
5. Push the plunger in slightly to force the air bubbles out of the syringe into the bottle.
6. Remove the syringe and check to make sure you've gotten the correct amount of units of insulin.
7. Pinch and pull up your skin at the injection site you've

chosen, making sure it is fatty tissue instead of muscle.

8. Take the syringe, push the needle straight into your skin, and depress the plunger slowly and evenly.
9. Dispose of the needle properly.

There are some recent developments in insulin injections. The *jet injector* is a needle-free, pressurized jet injector that delivers insulin directly to your bloodstream in a tiny stream. *Insulin pens* look like fountain pens and contain insulin. With these pens, you don't need to carry around syringes and vials. *Insulin pumps* are worn all day and all night and introduce insulin to your body at a slow pace through a plastic tube, which is inserted through your skin. Researchers are currently exploring ways to deliver insulin to your bloodstream through *nasal sprays*. Also, *pancreas transplantation* may someday replace insulin injection for some patients. This is a process by which the faulty insulin-producing cells in your pancreas would be replaced with new ones, taken from a human donor.

Control your diabetes through diet

Eating right is a good thing. If you have diabetes, try not to view changing your diet as a punishment. If so, everyone should be punished. Not only will instituting a good diet and exercise program help you to control your diabetes, it will also make you feel better. Get your family and friends to adopt a healthy lifestyle along with you. Having their support will also make maintaining your healthy lifestyle easier.

Because patients with diabetes commonly suffer from heart disease and high blood pressure, your nutrition plan must take all three of these conditions into account. If you are diabetic, your diet should be high in complex carbohydrates such as breads, beans, pasta, potatoes, fruits and other vegetables. These types of foods are good because they raise your energy level for a longer period of time than simple carbohydrates, such as the sugars in candy and cake. Your body has a hard time producing enough insulin to burn sweets. Since a Type I diabetic produces little or no insulin, you can see why you should stay away from simple carbohydrates, like those in desserts.

While fruits are good for you to eat, be careful. Natural sugar, or fructose, which is found in fruits, can increase your blood sugar level. If you are diabetic, it's okay for you to eat fruits and drink fruit juices, but be strict with yourself about limiting your fruit intake to the amounts you have been allotted by your nutritionist or diabetes educator. Always be aware of how much is too much. It can be a matter of life or death.

As a diabetic, you should also limit your fat and cholesterol intake. Fats and cholesterols can attach to the inside walls of your arteries, making it difficult for your blood to circulate. This, in turn, can lead to a decrease in blood flowing to your vital organs, as well as heart disease, kidney failure or a stroke. In cases of extremely poor circulation, it's sometimes necessary to amputate diabetics' toes, feet and/or legs. Since diabetics are already at a high risk for these problems, lessen your chances of these complications by decreasing your intake of fat and cholesterol. For more information on cholesterol, refer to Chapter Two and Chapter Four in this book.

The International Diabetic Center recommends the following guidelines to help you reduce the total fat in your diet. (All of these are discussed in greater detail in Chapter Two.)

- Limit meat portion sizes. Try to limit yourself to six ounces of meat per day.
- Use lean meats, such as fish and poultry. Choose meats that contain less than three grams of fat per ounce.
- Avoid high-fat meats, such as sausage, frankfurters, prime cuts of meats, luncheon meats and organ meats (for example, chitlins and liver).
- Cook to get rid of as much fat as possible. Broil, bake and boil foods instead of frying them, and remove fat from meats before making gravies and sauces.
- Use skim milk. If you now drink whole milk, gradually change from 2% to 1% milk, and then to skim milk.
- Use a margarine with a liquid vegetable oil as the first ingredient. Tub margarine contains more unsaturated fat than stick margarine. (See Chapter Two for a more detailed comparison of saturated and unsaturated fats.)
- Use liquid vegetable oils whenever possible.
- Limit your intake of eggs to three per week, at the most. Try to eat egg whites instead of egg yolks.
- Use low-fat or no-fat dairy products. Substitute low-fat or no-fat yogurt for cream and mayonnaise. Select cheeses with less than five grams of fat per ounce.
- There are more than 1,500 modified-fat products available in grocery stores today. Whenever possible, try to find a low-fat or fat-free alternative to the foods you like to eat.

Many of the dietary guidelines that we have recommended are important for all people, not just diabetics. For additional suggestions on how to eat a healthy diet, refer to Chapter Two. It's also important for you to realize that for the diabetic, what and how much you eat can have life-threatening implications. In addition to reducing fat, it's important for you to reduce your salt intake, since high levels of salt increase your risk of developing high blood pressure, for which, as a diabetic, you are at a high risk. (See Chapter Three for more information about how to lower your blood pressure.)

Develop your personal meal plan

Get involved in your meal planning. If you have diabetes, it is dangerous to simply "pick something up" at mealtime. Fast food is not a good idea for anyone, since it is high in calories, sugar, salt and cholesterol. Yet, for the diabetic, it is especially hazardous. Mealtime doesn't have to be a burden—it just takes getting used to. Remember, the ideal diet for a diabetic is the ideal diet for everyone. Look at being diabetic as being forced into living a more healthy lifestyle. Every diabetic faces a variety of problems, and each case should be handled individually. Your nutritionist or registered dietitian will help you devise a meal plan that's right for you. Health care specialists are learning more about diabetes daily, and current information can make your meal planning more flexible and enjoyable. Although you may feel limited in your choices, there are actually plenty of foods out there that you can eat.

The key to the diabetic diet is balance. You should stay on a relatively routine schedule because your diet is adjusted to your insulin intake, which should be relatively stable. Never skip a meal while taking insulin, or you could upset your body's balance. If you are unable to eat lunch at your regular time, eat a snack to keep you going until your meal is served. You don't want your blood glucose to drop too low at any time. A good balance between your diet and insulin will mean your body is processing your food at the same time the insulin in your body is peaking, or working the hardest.

Don't eat too much. This is common sense for everyone, not just diabetics. If you're overweight (Type II diabetics are more prone to being overweight than non-diabetics), losing some pounds could help you decrease the amount of insulin you have to take every day. Your doctor or registered dietitian should take your weight into consideration when they design your personal diet. Two sample meal plans are included in this chapter.

Changing your eating habits is one of the hardest lessons you may have to learn. This is especially true for black men, because many foods that are traditionally African-American are high in fat and salt. When we work to change our eating habits, we're combating hundreds of years of history and tradition. You've learned your eating habits over a lifetime, so you won't be able to change them in a day, a week or a month. You'll need to be patient with yourself and change them gradually.

Since you must become aware of your eating habits before you can change them, make an effort to record everything you eat and drink; how long it takes to eat your meals, including snacks; where you eat; with whom you eat; what else you were doing while you were eating; and how hungry you were. If you keep accurate records, you'll see patterns emerging. For instance, you'll know

Carbohydrate: 149 g   49% of total calories
Protein: 61 g   20% of total calories
Fat: 42 g   31% of total calories

These 2 menus show some of the ways the exchange lists can be used to add variety to your meals. Use the exchange lists to plan your own menus.

SAMPLE MENU 1	SAMPLE MENU 2

BREAKFAST

½ cup bran flakes cereal	½ bagel (whole wheat or pumpernickel)
½ banana	
8 oz skim or 1% milk	¾ cup mandarin oranges, drained and mixed with
	1 cup lemon nonfat yogurt

LUNCH

1 slice whole wheat bread	1 slice rye bread
2 oz lean ham	2 oz turkey breast
Carrot sticks and radishes	Sliced tomato, lettuce on sandwich
1 apple	2 fresh plums
1 Tbsp reduced-calorie mayonnaise	1 Tbsp reduced-calorie mayonnaise
OR 1 tsp margarine	

DINNER

1 small dinner roll	1 small dinner roll
⅓ cup brown rice	1 ear (6″) corn on cob
2 oz baked chicken	2 oz flank steak, broiled or grilled
½ cup cooked broccoli	½ cup green beans
1¼ cup strawberries	1 cup cantaloupe/honeydew melon salad
1 tsp margarine	

1 Tbsp regular salad dressing	1 tsp margarine for corn
Green salad	1 Tbsp slivered almonds for green beans

EVENING SNACK

3 graham cracker squares	1 oz (1½ cups) puffed wheat or rice cereal
8 oz skim or 1% milk	8 oz skim or 1% milk

FIGURE 5A

1,200-calorie meal plan.
Reprinted with permission from Eli Lilly & Company, 1992, *Managing Your Diabetes.*

just how many times you went to that fast food restaurant because you were in a hurry. Or, how many times you drank a glass of wine or a can of beer just to be sociable.

The second stage of this new program may be the most difficult. Now, you must avoid situations where your eating problems occur. Try to find snack substitutes, such as low-fat crackers (with less than two grams of fat per serving), raw vegetables and fresh fruits. Avoid walking past your favorite neighborhood candy store. Even if it takes a little longer for you to get home, the exercise will make you feel better.

If you can't avoid certain food-tempting situations, then implement a plan to eliminate problems before you're tempted into furthering them. If you do your own grocery shopping, make a shopping list and stick to it. Never go shopping on an empty stomach. While meal

Carbohydrate: 246 g 48% of total calories
Protein: 99 g 20% of total calories
Fat: 72 g 32% of total calories

These 2 menus show some of the ways the exchange lists can be used to add variety to your meals. Use the exchange lists to plan your own menus.

SAMPLE MENU 1	**SAMPLE MENU 2**

BREAKFAST

½ cup bran flakes cereal	1 bagel (whole wheat or pumpernickel)
1 slice whole wheat toast	
½ banana	¾ cup mandarin oranges, drained and mixed with
8 oz skim or 1% milk	
1 tsp margarine	1 cup lemon nonfat yogurt
	1 Tbsp cream cheese

LUNCH

2 slices whole wheat bread	2 slices rye bread
½ cup noodles in broth	3 graham cracker squares
2 oz lean ham	2 oz turkey breast
Carrot sticks and radishes	Sliced tomato, lettuce on sandwich
1 apple	2 fresh plums
8 oz skim or 1% milk	8 oz skim or 1% milk
2 Tbsp reduced-calorie mayonnaise	2 Tbsp reduced-calorie mayonnaise
OR 2 tsp margarine	

AFTERNOON SNACK

¾ oz pretzels	8 animal crackers

SAMPLE MENU 1	SAMPLE MENU 2
DINNER	
1 small dinner roll	1 small dinner roll
⅓ cup brown rice	1 ear (6″) corn on cob
4 oz baked chicken	4 oz flank steak, broiled or grilled
1 cup cooked carrots	½ cup green beans
1¼ cup strawberries	½ cup mushrooms, sauteed in 1
2 tsp margarine	tsp margarine
1 Tbsp regular salad dressing	1 cup cantaloupe/honeydew melon
Green salad	salad
	1 tsp margarine for corn
	1 Tbsp slivered almonds for green beans
EVENING SNACK	
3 graham cracker squares	1 oz (1½ cups) puffed wheat or rice
15 grapes	cereal
8 oz skim or 1% milk	½ banana
	8 oz skim or 1% milk

FIGURE 5B

2,000-calorie meal plan.
Reprinted with permission from Eli Lilly & Company, 1992, *Managing Your Diabetes.*

planning takes a little more time and effort, ultimately, the benefits will be worth it.

When you go to parties or restaurants, think ahead about what you're going to eat or order. Order first so you are not tempted by choices of the other members of your party. You'll probably notice that others will begin to adopt your healthy eating habits. Try to leave a little food on your plate at the end of a meal and, when you've eaten as much as you want, don't let anyone persuade you to "just take one more little bite." If you're sincere in your efforts to control your eating habits, you will succeed.

Jack exercises regularly

Deborah never knew her godfather to be overweight. At the age of 62, he was in great shape and he kept his weight in control by exercising. Jack either walked or rode his bike 30 minutes every day. It was something he lived by. If it rained, he rode his stationary bicycle in the house. During the cold winter months, Jack often walked in one of the local malls. He told Deborah that if it wasn't for exercise, he wouldn't feel nearly as good as he did every day. Deborah had never before realized that Jack's exercise was a major part of his diabetes treatment.

The benefits of regular exercise

If you are a diabetic, exercise is especially good for you. While food increases your blood sugar level, exercise decreases it by increasing your body's sensitivity to insulin. Aerobic exercise, such as walking, jogging, biking or swimming, is the best exercise for general fitness and for controlling your blood glucose level.

What complications can I develop if I have diabetes?

The longer you have uncontrolled diabetes, the more likely it is that you'll develop complications. Some of the major complications you can develop are discussed below.

Your risk of developing heart disease and stroke increases

If you are diabetic, you have a two to four times higher risk of suffering heart disease and stroke. Fat and cholesterol are more likely to deposit on the walls of your blood vessels, and when the blood vessels that nourish your heart become clogged, a heart attack can occur. If the arteries leading to your brain become blocked, a stroke can occur because the blockage keeps your brain from receiving oxygen and nutrients. (For more information about heart disease and stroke, see Chapter Four.)

You can lose your sight

Diabetes is the leading cause of blindness in the United States. Approximately 12,000 diabetics lose their sight each year. In fact, if you have diabetes for 15 years or more, you are likely to develop some sort of damage to blood vessels in your eye. Sometimes, the small blood vessels in the back of your eye will suffer from damage and changes. Mild blood vessel changes are called background retinopathy.

If you have diabetes, you may also have cataracts, glaucoma or swelling in the back of your eyes. All these problems can affect your vision and may lead to blindness. Most often, early eye disease has no symptoms, which is why an annual visit to your eye doctor is extremely important, so that treatment can be administered before irreparable damage occurs.

You are at a greater risk of developing kidney disease

Your kidneys can also be affected by damage to your small blood vessels. Diabetic disease of the kidneys is called "diabetic nephropathy." According to the Juvenile Diabetes Foundation International and The Diabetes Research Foundation, approximately 30 percent of new dialysis patients have diabetes-caused kidney failure. Your doctor can tell if you have diabetic kidney disease, first by detecting elevated protein in your urine, which indicates that your kidneys are damaged. When you lose too much protein through your urine, your ankles swell and fluids can build up in your lungs. Advanced diabetic kidney disease is usually accompanied by high blood pressure. If you can control your high blood pressure, you are taking a positive step toward controlling diabetic kidney disease. (See Chapter Eight for more information about kidney disease.)

You may experience nerve damage

Neuropathy, or nerve damage, is the least understood of all the small blood vessel complications of diabetes. When the small blood vessels around your nerves become damaged by high blood glucose levels, your nerves aren't able to function properly. This damage dulls the sensitivity of your nerve endings. Diabetic neuropathy can affect any nerve system in your body, but is most commonly seen in the feet and lower legs.

If you suffer from neuropathy, it can lead to a loss of

sensation in your feet, which becomes a problem if you suffer an injury or infection and don't know it. If the nerves in your feet are severely damaged, you can develop gangrene, which can spread throughout your feet and legs, requiring amputation. So if you are a diabetic, make it part of your daily routine to check your feet and legs for possible cuts or infections.

You can become impotent

Another major complication of diabetes is impotence. Impotence develops slowly over many months or years. Erections become softer and less frequent until there is a total inability to achieve erection. There are many new methods of treatment that may make erection and intercourse possible. If you are experiencing impotence, consult your health care professional or a urologist about available options.

Your risk of developing skin and teeth problems increases

People with diabetes are more prone to have skin and teeth disease than others. Periodontal disease is a disease of the gums that is more common in diabetics than others, and is the main reason why people lose their teeth when they get older. Consult your dentist about ways to best prevent periodontal disease from happening to you.

You may experience hypoglycemia

Hypoglycemia simply means low blood sugar, and is sometimes called an insulin reaction. This can occur because of intense activity, going without a meal or from taking too much insulin. Symptoms of hypoglycemia can include trembling, sweating, hunger and a rapid heart-beat. If you are diabetic, these symptoms may mean you are experiencing an emergency. You must replace sugar in your body by taking concentrated sugar. It is always a good idea to keep glucose tablets or hard candy, such as Life Savers, with you at all times in case this should ever happen to you or someone you know.

DCCT study

The good news is that the majority of these complications may be delayed or avoided by keeping tight control over your blood sugar. A recently concluded governmental study, the Diabetes Complications Control Trial (DCCT), demonstrated that the complications of diabetes (mentioned above) can be reduced up to 60 percent with tight blood sugar control. The study proves even further the importance of following the guidelines outlined in this chapter to prevent diabetes-related complications from happening to you.

Conclusion

How diabetes affects your life is up to you. It only takes about ten minutes each day to take care of a diabetic condition, and most diabetics take care of it in even less time than that. If you are diabetic, you now have the information you need to control unnecessary complications. You're also part of a well-educated team of health care providers. Your fellow teammates can help you to approach each aspect of your disease and to tackle any challenges that may arise. Get a complete physical, check your blood sugar level regularly, plan your meals, watch your weight and exercise regularly. By following these simple guidelines, like many other diabetics, you, too, can grow old gracefully with diabetes.

Resources

American Association of Diabetes Educators
444 N. Michigan Avenue
Suite 1240
Chicago, IL 60611
(312) 662-1700
Fax (312) 644-2233

(This is an organization of health professionals who provide diabetes education for patients. Call or fax them to obtain a nationwide directory of diabetes educators.)

American Diabetes Association
1660 Duke Street
Alexandria, VA 22314
(800) 232-3472

(The Association gives information and referrals, and has quarterly journals and a newsletter. There is a fee for some publications.)

Juvenile Diabetes Foundation International
229 Peachtree Street, N.E.
Caine Tower, Suite 1202
Atlanta, GA 30303
(404) 688-2646

National Diabetes Information Clearinghouse
(301) 645-3327

(The Clearinghouse offers brochures and fact sheets, newsletters, and an on-line database.)

6

Cancer

Lonnie's story

Lonnie, an author, was the type of man everyone envied. He was happily married, had six children and appeared to everyone to have a "perfect life." He'd written twenty books and his success had been great. But the constant threat of deadlines had made Lonnie's previously easygoing life stressful. He started smoking more often, which he rationalized away as a stress-reliever. With all the social functions he was invited to attend as a successful novelist, he began drinking more alcohol.

One winter, Lonnie developed a nagging cough, which he first simply attributed to a winter cold. When it lingered, he blamed it on allergies. Finally, a few months later, he went to a doctor to have it checked. A chest x-ray revealed a small, isolated white spot—the size of a quarter—in Lonnie's lungs. He had cancer.

Most of us have known someone with cancer. When we hear the word, we instantly feel fear. Perhaps that's because cancer is commonly misperceived as a death sentence. Many people don't realize that 50 percent of all cancer patients have more than a five-year survival rate, and many are cured! But what determines who is cured and who is not? What is cancer? And how can you prevent it from happening to you?

What causes cancer?

There are many different risk factors for developing cancer. Most common is the aging process. Everyone's risk of cancer is increasing because, as a population, we are living longer. Many people diagnosed with cancer may have no idea what caused it. In reality, the disease may be caused by an accumulation of different factors over your lifetime. Cancer is becoming more common among older individuals. This phenomenon will probably continue to increase, especially as heart disease mortality declines and the average life span increases.

Because the most common cause of cancer is living, it's important to know how to live a preventative lifestyle. We already discussed prevention in Chapter Two, but there are also specific preventive measures you can take to reduce your risk of cancer. For example, fruits and vegetables have emerged as having a strong protective effect against many cancers. A high-fiber diet can also help prevent cancer by limiting the amount of time carcinogens remain in your body. By eating these foods throughout your lifetime, you may be making large strides against contracting cancer later in life. Avoiding alcohol can also help you to prevent many common cancers, such as cancers of the esophagus, larynx, mouth and throat.

The Seventh Day Adventists, a religious group, espouse a strictly vegetarian diet that contains great amounts of fruit, vegetables and whole grains. They also avoid alcohol, tea and coffee. As a population, they have been recorded to have one-half the rate of cancer of the general population.[1]

Another cause of cancer is exposure to chemicals called carcinogens. Although you may not feel at risk, carcinogens often work silently, altering the DNA (deoxyribonucleic acid that controls cell function) in each cell without your even knowing it. Once cells are altered and become cancerous, they reproduce much more rapidly than normal cells. Growth can be uncontrollable, spreading rapidly to other parts of your body, often in the form of tumors.

Smoke contains carcinogens that increase your risk of lung cancer. If you smoke, quit—it's the most effective way to prevent the disease. Other carcinogens may not always be so easily recognized or avoided. For example, for many years asbestos was commonly found in many work environments. It was only when employees began to be diagnosed with cancer that this substance was later identified as a carcinogen. (See the Appendix for information on carcinogens in the workplace.)

Several government agencies now protect us from carcinogens in the workplace. These include the Occupational Safety and Health Administration (OSHA) and the National Institute of Occupational Safety (NIOS). The Food and Drug Administration (FDA) identifies carcinogens in drug and food additives and the Environmental Protection Agency (EPA) attempts to control carcinogens in our air and water.

Regardless of how careful you are about avoiding carcinogens, everyone is at risk. That risk may even be increased further if someone in your family had cancer. For Lonnie, as with many cancer patients, a number of factors probably contributed to his disease. For example, high levels of stress may have lowered his immune system, or his resistance to disease. "Social drinking" could have changed the balance in his cells, making him more vulnerable to cancer. Cigarette smoke alone contains forty known carcinogens and accounts for approximately 30 percent of all cancer deaths!

Eating "party food" may also have contributed to Lonnie's cancer. Poor diet accounts for approximately 35 percent of cancer deaths. Whether you're fighting cancer or simply working for prevention, it's important to strive for balance and health in all areas of your life. (See Chapter Two for more information about making lifestyle changes.)

Why are blacks more likely to die of cancer than whites?

So now we've established some of the causes of cancer, but that doesn't explain the increased risk of cancer-related deaths in black Americans. Blacks have a much higher adjusted cancer death rate than whites, and their average survival time is significantly shorter. In 1987, 288 out of 100,000 black males and 158 out of 100,000 white males died from cancer. For black females, the rate was 132 per 100,000 versus 110 per 100,000 for white females.[2]

There are many causes for these inequalities. While some hereditary cancers seem to be more common among blacks, most cancers, such as lung cancer, are a direct result of environmental and lifestyle factors. By learning how to take better care of ourselves, we may be able to reverse some of the statistics. These inequalities may also be due to late diagnosis. Many cancers are more frequently diagnosed in a localized stage among whites than among blacks. This means that by the time a black man's cancer has been diagnosed by a doctor, it may already have spread too much to be treated effectively. Early detection and timely treatment can increase your chance of survival. Many blacks are at a distinct disadvantage because of poverty, lack of access to medical care and discrimination. Clearly, if we were able to make environmental and social changes *as well as* improvements in our own knowledge and awareness of medicine and preventive strategies, rates of death from cancer would radically decrease among black men.

There are indications that if a person believes he or she can get well, his or her chance of being cured may increase. National surveys indicate that blacks overestimate the deadliness of cancer and underestimate cancer prevalence in their population. Additionally, blacks are less knowledgeable about cancer-related warning signs and screening methods than whites. Even with early detection, if blacks are more pessimistic about the curability of cancer than other racial groups, it could be we're seeing this lack of information play itself out as a broad social phenomenon.

But what can we do about it? "Knowledge, attitudes and practices are important to understanding factors that relate to people seeking care for cancer," according to the *Report of the Secretary on Black Minority Welfare and Health*. The differences between the awareness and outlook of blacks and whites may help to explain the longer delay in seeking diagnosis and treatment among blacks and the greater occurrence of more advanced stages of cancer.

Because cancer may be entirely avoidable with proper

diet, a healthy lifestyle and by reducing a variety of environmental risks, the first step in eradicating these racial discrepancies is education. Prevention is the only cure with a 100 percent guarantee. Early detection can also greatly increase your chance of being cured. By getting frequent checkups and specifically requesting diagnostic tests for cancer, you can help your doctor determine if you have cancer, or if you are at risk. You can also detect cancer on your own. Make it a habit to frequently check your body for abnormalities. If you notice any change in your energy level or if you see or feel spots, lumps or physical symptoms that seem suspicious, ask your doctor about them. Later in this chapter, we will discuss common signs of cancer you should watch for.

Lonnie is diagnosed

Lonnie fortunately went to the doctor before his cancer had a chance to spread. His doctor told him he was very lucky—it is very rare for lung cancer to be detected early. He prescribed surgery to remove Lonnie's cancer, as well as chemotherapy to kill any remaining cancer cells. In addition to this treatment, Lonnie started making changes in his lifestyle. The first major change he knew he had to make was to stop smoking. Lonnie figured he was probably doing other things that put him at risk for the disease, so he requested information from the American Cancer Society.

As Lonnie was taking his roller coaster ride toward the elimination of smoking in his life, he learned that he was an addict. Instead of being hooked on cocaine, marijuana, crack or heroin, he was hooked on nicotine.

Tobacco-related cancers account for approximately 45 percent of new cancer cases in black males, 25 percent in black females. These cancers also account for approximately 37 percent of cancer deaths in black males and 20 percent in black females.[3] With prevention and by eliminating tobacco use, all of these deaths could be avoided. Although the percentage of people who smoke is decreasing each year, approximately 46 million American adults still smoke.[4] If you smoke, stop. (For more information about how to quit smoking, see Chapter Two.)

Cancer of the Lung

Singer and jazz pianist Nat "King" Cole began his career in the late 1930s as the leader of the King Cole Trio. Later, his velvet voice made him a musical legend. Cole, one of the first blacks to successfully cross over and appeal to white audiences, realized late in his life the dangers of smoking and tried to warn others. In his biography, written by James Haskins with Kathleen Benson, it says that Cole "talked about how important it was to warn children against smoking and expressed interest in doing advertisements for the American Cancer Society." Cole, a smoker, died from lung cancer shortly after making the statement.

Smoke irritates the lining of your bronchi (the main airways of your lungs), which can cause the cilia (hair-like structures that filter the air entering the lungs) to disappear. Extra mucus, produced to make up for the lack of cilia, causes the coughing experienced by most smokers. If you have a persistent cough, blood-streaked sputum, chest pain, recurring pneumonia or bronchitis, see your doctor immediately. If you are diagnosed with cancer, your doctor can work with you to determine the most appropriate treatment. (For more information on how to break yourself of addictions, see Chapter Two on taking control, and Chapter Ten on substance abuse.)

Prevention and early detection

Lung cancer, as mentioned before, is a very common cancer among black males. But there are many forms of cancer, often with unique methods of prevention and recommended treatment. A high-fiber and low-fat diet, regular exercise and reduced levels of stress are simple ways you can prevent or control the spread of most cancers. In specific types, as you'll see, these prevention methods can be especially effective.

Early detection also greatly increases your chance of being cured. Watch your body closely, day by day, for any changes that may indicate a problem. In the early stages of many cancers you may not experience any symptoms. Often, symptoms associated with cancer are more commonly seen when the disease has reached a more advanced stage. Because of that, it's important to see your doctor for regular checkups.

According to the American Cancer Society, there are seven general warning signs of cancer:

1. Change in bowel or bladder habits
2. A sore throat that does not heal
3. Unusual bleeding or discharge from the genital, urinary or digestive tract
4. Thickening or a lump in a breast or elsewhere
5. Indigestion or difficulty swallowing
6. Obvious change in a wart or mole
7. Nagging cough or hoarseness[5]

If you notice any of these symptoms, consult your physician immediately.

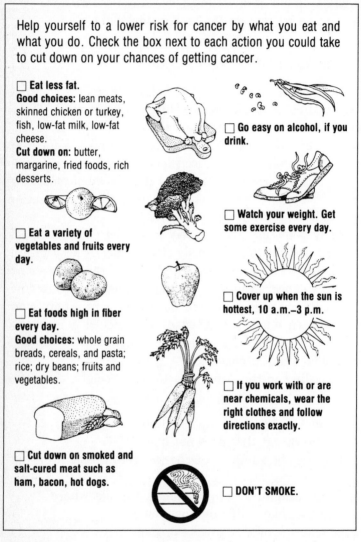

Help yourself to a lower risk for cancer by what you eat and what you do. Check the box next to each action you could take to cut down on your chances of getting cancer.

☐ **Eat less fat.**
Good choices: lean meats, skinned chicken or turkey, fish, low-fat milk, low-fat cheese.
Cut down on: butter, margarine, fried foods, rich desserts.

☐ **Eat a variety of vegetables and fruits every day.**

☐ **Eat foods high in fiber every day.**
Good choices: whole grain breads, cereals, and pasta; rice; dry beans; fruits and vegetables.

☐ **Cut down on smoked and salt-cured meat such as ham, bacon, hot dogs.**

☐ **Go easy on alcohol, if you drink.**

☐ **Watch your weight. Get some exercise every day.**

☐ **Cover up when the sun is hottest, 10 a.m.–3 p.m.**

☐ **If you work with or are near chemicals, wear the right clothes and follow directions exactly.**

☐ **DON'T SMOKE.**

FIGURE 6A

9 steps to a healthier life with less risk of cancer.
Reprinted with permission from the American Cancer Society pamphlet titled "Choice or Chance."

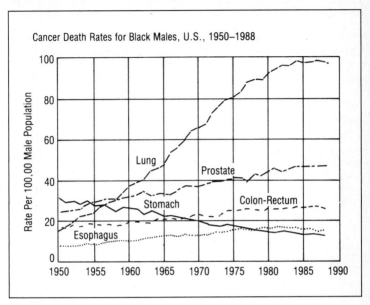

Cancer Death Rates for Black Males, U.S., 1950–1988

FIGURE 6B

Cancer mortality rates for black males, U.S., 1950–1988.
Reprinted with permission from the American Cancer Society booklet titled "Cancer Facts and Figures for Minority Americans, 1991."

Other common cancers in black males

There are many cancers that are common among black men. Following are some of these, beginning with those with the highest rates of related deaths for black males in the U.S. But this is only a start. If you or a loved one is seeking to prevent or cure a specific cancer, become as educated as possible so that you are fully armed against the disease. The end of this chapter lists several resources you can use to begin your search.

Cancer Site	Black Males	Black Females	American Indian	Chinese	Japanese	Hispanic*
All sites	31,452	24,112	1,318	1,425	1,124	13,538
Oral cavity	939	312	23	62	14	209
Esophagus	1,524	523	20	28	29	257
Stomach	1,390	859	54	86	139	793
Colon & rectum	2,765	3,080	131	169	164	1,327
Liver & other biliary	791	568	85	153	53	754
Pancreas	1,403	1,551	74	68	84	690
Lung (male)	10,457	—	221	239	139	1,789
Lung (female)	—	4,246	118	134	78	800
Breast (female)	—	4,403	90	62	78	1,115
Cervix uteri	—	1,049	31	19	10	274
Other uterus	—	873	12	22	9	159
Ovary	—	901	26	31	34	365
Prostate	4,785	—	71	40	36	689
Bladder	484	369	14	8	26	224
Kidney	525	363	46	14	18	334
Brain & CNS	335	299	30	22	10	373
Lymphoma	750	558	40	45	52	722
Leukemia	868	672	45	50	37	645
Multiple myeloma	684	703	30	13	8	271

* Persons classified as Hispanic origin on death certificates may be of any race. Hispanic deaths in 1989 were reported in 44 states and the District of Columbia. Hispanic deaths in the following six states are not included: Connecticut, Louisiana, Maryland, New Hampshire, Oklahoma, and Virginia. In 1980, the reporting areas accounted for about 97% of the Hispanic population in the United States. Caution should be exercised in generalizing this mortality data to the entire United States Hispanic population.

Available on reproduction sheet (5005.93)

FIGURE 6C

Cancer mortality rates by race in U.S., 1989.
Reprinted with permission from the American Cancer Society booklet titled "Cancer Facts and Figures for Minority Americans, 1991."

Cancer Site	Black Males
All sites	31,452
Oral cavity	939
Esophagus	1,524
Stomach	1,390
Colon & rectum	2,765
Liver & other biliary	791
Pancreas	1,403
Lung	10,457
Prostate	4,785
Bladder	484
Kidney	525
Brain & CNS	335
Lymphoma	750
Leukemia	868
Multiple myeloma	684

FIGURE 6D

Number of cancer deaths for black men in U.S., 1989.
Reprinted with permission from the American Cancer Society booklet titled "Cancer Facts and Figures," 1993, p. 19.

PROSTATE CANCER

Incidence: Prostate cancer is the most common cancer among black men. Every man is at risk for this disease. Make sure you pay close attention to the prevention and early detection strategies mentioned here. Never skip or delay an annual checkup and ask your doctor any questions you may have about this cancer.

In 1991, 15,000 new cases of prostate cancer were reported among black men. In the same year, 5,000 black men died of the disease. Between 1986 and 1990, 38.5

more black than white men were diagnosed with, and 27.6 more black than white men died of, this cancer, per 100,000.

It is difficult to determine whether the high rate of prostate cancer among black Americans is due to genetic or environmental factors. Some medical experts suggest that eating a diet high in fat content may be a contributing factor for this disease. The inequalities between black and white men when it comes to this disease may also stem from differences in access to medical care, early detection and awareness of treatment strategies.

Prevention: New research shows a healthy diet with lots of fruits and vegetables and low in alcohol may help prevent this cancer. No other prevention methods are known, although exposure to cadmium in the workplace may be a cause.

Warning signs: Weak or interrupted urine flow; difficulty urinating; the need to urinate frequently; pain in the lower back, pelvis or upper thighs; blood in urine; and painful ejaculations are symptoms.

Detection: Every man over 40 should have a digital rectal examination as part of his regular annual physical checkup. This test can help detect prostate cancer early. Also, men over 50 should have annual prostate-specific antigen blood testing. If the results of either of these tests seem suspicious, a new technique known as transrectal ultrasound can be used to reveal cancers that are too small to be detected through a physical exam.

Treatment: Surgery and chemotherapy are often used to treat this cancer. Estrogen supplements may also be prescribed to limit cancer growth.

CANCER OF THE COLON AND RECTUM

Incidence: In 1991, 6,800 new cases of colon and rectum cancer were reported among black men. In the same year, 2,900 black men died of these diseases. Between 1986 and 1990, .3 more black than white men were diagnosed with, and 4.2 more black than white men died of, this cancer, per 100,000.

From these statistics, you can see that being black does not necessarily put you at greater risk for these diseases than if you were white. However, being black does seem to have a great effect on whether or not you will survive the cancers. Because colon or rectum cancers are so closely linked to diet, one cause for this inequality may be a diet high in fat and low in fiber.

Prevention: A high-fiber diet, including fruits, grains and vegetables, can help prevent colon cancer. This reduces the concentration of carcinogens in your colon because bowel movements are more frequent.

Warning signs: Rectal bleeding and blood in the stool are symptoms.

Detection: After age 40, ask your doctor for a digital rectal exam, stool blood test and rectum and lower colon exam (flexible sigmoidoscopic) every three to five years. If you are older than 50, ask about a colonoscopic exam. This involves a lighted instrument, a colonoscope, which can view the entire colon.

Treatment: Surgery, chemotherapy or a combination of both can be effective treatments for this cancer, depending on the specific type of cancer and its stage.

CANCER OF THE ESOPHAGUS

Incidence: In 1991, 2,100 new cases of esophageal cancer were reported among black men. In the same year, 1,500 black men died of the disease. Between 1986 and 1990, out of a sample of 100,000, 13 more black than white men were diagnosed with, and 10.3 more black than white men died of this cancer. The difference in the traditional diets of blacks and whites may be one cause for this inequality.

Prevention: To prevent this cancer, *avoid alcohol* and fatty, processed foods. Eat a balanced diet, full of fresh fruits and vegetables.

Warning signs: Symptoms can be difficulty in swallowing or a brief pain from behind the breastbone or esophageal area when swallowing.

Detection: A special X ray called a barium swallow can be used to detect cancer of the esophagus. This involves drinking a chalklike liquid that contains barium, which coats the esophagus walls and allows your physician to see the esophagus more clearly. Your doctor may also place a gastroscope (tube) down your throat for better detection.

Treatment: Several treatments are commonly used for cancer of the esophagus, depending on its stage. Surgery is the most common.

CANCER OF THE PANCREAS

Incidence: In 1991, 1,800 new cases of pancreatic cancer were reported among black men. In the same year, 1,400 black men died of the disease. Between 1986 and 1990, out of a sample of 100,000, 5 more black than white men were diagnosed with, and 4.5 more black than white men died of this cancer. These inequalities may stem from differences in traditional diets among blacks and whites and lifestyle habits, such as the tendency among blacks to smoke more menthol cigarettes than whites.

Prevention: Don't smoke; eat a high-fiber, low-fat diet.

Warning signs: Symptoms may not occur until the cancer is in advanced stages. Warning signals include abdominal pain, which may spread to the back; a loss of appetite, nausea and drastic weight loss or weakness.

Detection: Ultrasound imaging and computerized tomography (CT) scans are being tried to detect the disease earlier. Very little is known about causes or methods of prevention.

Treatment: Chemotherapy and surgery are often used.

CANCER OF THE STOMACH

Incidence: In 1991, 2,100 new cases of stomach cancer were reported among black men. In the same year, 1,300 black men died of the disease. Between 1986 and 1990, out of a sample of 100,000, 8.6 more black than white men were diagnosed with, and 7.3 more black than white men died of, this cancer. Again, the difference in the traditional diets of blacks and whites may be one cause for this inequality.

Prevention: Avoid cured and preserved foods with nitrites, such as frankfurters, beef jerky and smoked and aged meats. Nitrites are carcinogens that are contained in many foods.

Warning signs: Loss of appetite, heartburn, stomach pain or feeling full early in a meal can be signs of stomach cancer. If symptoms last for longer than one month, consult your physician.

Detection: Early detection of stomach cancer can be difficult.

Treatment: Removal of part or all of the stomach is a common treatment. If the cancer has spread and cannot be removed by surgery, chemotherapy may be used. Radiation (which is discussed later in this chapter) is rarely used in stomach cancer, since the amount of radiation necessary to kill stomach cancer cells is so high that there is danger of destroying healthy organs or tissues.

CANCER OF THE ORAL CAVITY AND PHARYNX

Incidence: In 1991, 2,900 new cases of oral cancer were reported among black men. In the same year, 875 black men died of the disease. Between 1986 and 1990, out of a sample of 100,000, 8.5 more black than white men were diagnosed with, and 5.2 more black than white men died of, these cancers. These inequalities may stem from differences in traditional diets among blacks and whites, and lifestyle habits, such as smoking menthol cigarettes, and drinking alcohol.

Prevention: *Avoid alcohol.* Don't smoke or use chewing tobacco; work to ensure that your home and work environments are smoke-free.

Warning signs: Signs of oral cancer are sores that bleed easily and don't heal, and difficulty in swallowing and chewing.

Detection: Make sure you have regular checkups with your dentist and doctor. Abnormal tissue changes can often be detected during regular examinations.

Treatment: If cancer is contained to single areas, such as the tongue, lips or gums, 76 percent can be treated successfully, with a five-year or greater survival rate. However, if the cancer has spread before detection, this percentage drops to 34 percent.

LEUKEMIAS

Incidence: In 1991, 1,300 new cases of leukemias were reported among black men. In the same year, 850 black men died of these diseases. Between 1986 and 1990, out of a sample of 100,000, 1.9 more white than black men were diagnosed with, and .6 more white than black men died of, these cancers. Because leukemia is hereditary, you are at increased risk for this disease if it runs in your family. Ask your relatives if your family has a history of this disease.

Prevention: No methods of prevention are known, except to avoid excessive exposure to toxic chemicals or known carcinogens.

Warning signs: Weight loss, repeated infections, fatigue, unusual paleness, bruising easily, and nosebleeds or hemorrhages are common symptoms.

Detection: Symptoms can seem to be those of less serious conditions. Blood tests and biopsy of the bone marrow can determine if what you have is actually leukemia.

Treatment: Chemotherapy, surgery and radiation therapy are all used to fight leukemias.

LYMPHOMA

Incidence: In 1991, 1,500 new cases of non-Hodgkin's lymphoma were reported among black men. In the same year, 650 black men died of the disease. Between 1986 and 1990, 7.3 more white than black men were diagnosed with, and 2.2 more white than black men died of, these cancers, per 100,000.

Prevention: Risk factors for lymphomas are largely unknown. What we do know is that if, for any reason, you are experiencing reduced function of your immune system or have been exposed to certain infectious agents, you may be at risk. If you had an organ transplant, you may be at increased risk, because your immune functions may be altered. Carrying HIV—the AIDS virus—can also be a risk factor of lymphoma. (See Chapter Nine for tips on how to prevent the virus.)

Warning signs: Symptoms of lymphoma are enlargement of glands, including the spleen, but no tenderness or pain.

Detection: No methods of early detection are known.

Treatment: Surgery, chemotherapy and radiation therapy have been used.[6]

Cancer treatments

Common cancer treatments are surgery, radiation therapy and chemotherapy. Other, newer medical therapies include neutron-capture, photo dynamic and hormonal drug therapies. In addition to these treatments, many non-medical alternative therapies are being researched by the medical community. Radical diet changes, positive imaging, increased exercise, humor and relaxation techniques may be helpful but these should be used in conjunction with, not as substitutes for, traditional therapies. Often, a patient's greatest chance of cure may include a combination of several of these methods.

Once your diagnosis has been confirmed, it is up to you, with help from your doctor, family members and trusted love ones, to determine your next move. Your treatment is a joint venture between you and your doctor. Take an active role in the decisions made regarding your health, and request that your doctor explain the benefits and consequences of each type of treatment recommended. Never hesitate to seek a second opinion.

Treating cancer with surgery

The oldest treatment for cancer is surgery, whereby a surgeon removes cancerous cell growth such as a tumor, while cutting away as little healthy tissue as possible. Surgery is a delicate treatment—if your surgeon removes too much healthy tissue, complications may occur. On the other hand, if too little cancer tissue is removed, you may not be cured.

More than one-third of all cancers spread in a slow, predictable manner. Only cancer that is confined to the tumor site or the regional lymph nodes can be totally removed by surgery. If cancer has spread throughout your body or to your vital organs, other treatments should be explored. All cancer patients must have periodic checkups for the rest of their lives. If the cancer has not recurred after five years, you are usually considered to be cured.

Treating cancer with radiation therapy

In order to destroy certain cancer cells, your doctor may also use highly active, invisible beams of energy called X rays or gamma rays. X rays are produced by machines, and gamma rays are given off by radioactive substances, such as cobalt, cesium, iridium and radium. When radioactive substances are used in the treatment of cancer, they may be housed in a machine that delivers their rays, or placed in a small container that is inserted into one of your body cavities or put directly into a tumor.

X rays can be neither seen nor felt, but they can attack cancer cells. Radiation therapy often cures cancer in two ways: by destroying cancer cells and by sterilizing cancer cells so that they can no longer reproduce. Some cancers are more sensitive than normal tissue to the destructive effects of X rays, such as cancer of the lymph nodes, cancer of the testicle and childhood cancers. In these cases, the doctor can irradiate cancer cells in large parts of the body without causing excessive damage to normal tissue.

Radiation is generally used only when the area to be treated is small. When cancer becomes widespread, radiation can seldom produce a cure, although it may be used to alleviate the symptoms that accompany cancer. X ray treatment is also used to treat cancers that cannot be surgically removed or cancers that are best not removed because they are vital to the patient's normal activities, such as in the vocal cords and tongue. In other cases, when your doctor is concerned that surgery may leave some cancer cells behind, radiation therapy may be used afterwards.

As in any treatment, don't rush into radiation therapy until all your questions and concerns have been answered and a program has been specifically designed to meet your individual needs. X rays always destroy some of your healthy cells along with your cancerous cells. The doctor's task is to destroy the cancer with a minimum of injury to your normal tissues. Normal cells can repair themselves more efficiently than cancer cells. For this reason, radiation sessions are spaced so that your healthy cells have time to heal.

If you're undergoing radiation therapy, you may experience some side effects in the area of the body being treated. For example, if your throat is being treated, you may experience a sore throat and difficulty in swallowing. If the area being treated is your bladder or rectum, you may experience frequent urination, cramps or diarrhea. Nausea is a side effect for those patients whose stomachs are being treated. However, in most instances, these side effects can be controlled with medication.

One out of every 20 patients experiences delayed side effects such as weakness, nausea, diarrhea, and vomiting from the radiation treatment. This can happen from six months after radiation therapy is discontinued, to many years later. Radiation of the ovaries or testes can also cause infertility. Very rarely does radiation cause new cancers. The success of radiation therapy cannot be determined by the speed at which a tumor shrinks. Slowly growing tumors shrink slowly, while fast-growing tumors shrink quickly.

Treating cancer with chemotherapy

The use of medication to fight cancer is called chemotherapy. Chemotherapy treatment is often given in periodic sessions during which various anticancer drugs are administered. Each type of drug works differently. For example, one drug may kill cancer cells by disrupting the process of cell division, another may prevent cells from making the nutrients that keep them alive, and still another may create hormonal conditions in your body that will not allow the cancer cells to survive. Any drug that kills cancer cells may kill some of your normal cells as well.

Chemotherapy is often used when cancerous cells have spread throughout your body and their locations cannot be precisely determined. Unlike surgery and radiation therapy, drugs can circulate throughout your entire body, killing the cancer cells missed by other treatments.

Some cancers can be cured by drugs alone. These may include: acute leukemia, cancer of the placenta, lymphoma and cancer of the testicle. Even when drugs cannot produce a cure, chemotherapy may still be useful, since drugs often extend the lives of patients. Drugs may be used during radiation therapy to improve a tumor's response to X rays. They may also be used for "adjuvant chemotherapy" after surgery, in which doctors use chemotherapy as a precautionary measure when they are uncertain if some cancer still remains. The drugs are intended to destroy cancerous cells that may be alive but undetected in the body.

Drugs used in chemotherapy can be administered in several ways. Some must be given orally, while others must be injected either under the skin or into a muscle. The most common types of chemotherapy drugs are given through a needle that is placed in a vein, an artery or the space surrounding the spinal cord. When a single drug can be administered in several ways, the doctor will choose the way best suited to the particular cancer, the prescribed dosage and your comfort.

Chemotherapy can be administered weekly, bimonthly or monthly, and for short periods of time may be administered daily. Most times, chemotherapy can be done on an outpatient basis, but sometimes you may have to be hospitalized.

Like all treatments, chemotherapy has its limitations. If this treatment is chosen, make sure your doctor explains the side effects. Because the drugs used may kill normal cells while acting on the cancerous ones, tissues may be damaged, especially those that are made of frequently dividing cells, such as the stomach and intestines, mucous membranes, hair follicles and bone marrow. Sometimes nausea, vomiting and diarrhea result from damage to the digestive tract; dryness and soreness of the mouth may occur from damage to the mucous membranes; also, hair loss may occur from damage to the hair follicles. When bone marrow is damaged, the marrow no longer supplies the blood with the necessary white blood cells, platelets and red blood cells, so that the body cannot properly control infection, bruising or fatigue. Certainly, if you suffer severe side effects from chemotherapeutic treatment, you should work with your physician to have the therapy adjusted.

Lonnie finds life after cancer

Since Lonnie's diagnosis, he's made some major changes in his lifestyle, in addition to undergoing chemotherapy and surgery. He's stopped smoking, eats healthy foods and exercises regularly. Ask him, though, and he'll tell you that all the changes were well worth the adjustment. It's been five years since his last treatment and, while he still goes to the doctor for regular checkups, as far as his doctor is concerned, Lonnie has had no recurrence of cancer.

Conclusion

As Lonnie learned, it is never too late to quit smoking or to change your diet to a healthier one. Even though cancer is often curable, it's best to make these lifestyle changes before it happens. Cancer prevention is only one of the benefits of healthy habits. By cutting down on your intake of fats, cholesterol, excessive calories and salt and by exercising regularly, you'll not only boost your immune system against disease, you'll feel better every day.

Resources

American Cancer Society
1599 Clifton Road, N.E.
Atlanta, GA 30329
(800) ACS-2345

(The Society offers information, programs and patient services.)

American Lung Association
1740 Broadway
New York, NY 10019-4374
(212) 315-8700

(The Association offers general information about lung cancer and how to quit smoking.)

Cancer Fax
(National Cancer Institute)
(301) 402-5874

(Fax your request for information about all different types of cancer and their treatment to this number. Your request will be fulfilled by fax.)

Cancer Research Institute
681 5th Avenue, 12th Floor
New York, NY 10022
(800) 99-CANCER

(You can receive information about and referrals to cancer studies by calling this 800 number. They will also answer questions and provide literature about your specific areas of interest.)

National Cancer Institute
9000 Rockville Pike
Building 31, Room 4A-18
Bethesda, MD 20892
(800) ACS-2345

(The Institute offers patient information and free brochures about diet, cancer prevention and treatment.)

Office on Smoking and Health
Centers for Disease Control
4770 Buford Highway, N.E.
Mail Stop K-50
Atlanta, GA 30341
404-488-5705

(This group offers information about tobacco control and statistics about quitting smoking.)

7

Sickle Cell Disease

Fletcher's story

Fletcher is a husky, dark-skinned 35-year-old man with a smile so wide that his face seems to disappear when he's really happy. He works for the florist in his local hospital delivering flowers. He loves his job, especially the fact that he is responsible for delivering a little bit of happiness into others' lives. If the patient he is visiting is awake, he never leaves without saying a few kind words. And if one of them seems especially lonely, he always takes time out of his busy day to sit down and start a conversation. Fletcher takes his job very seriously. If he thinks he can make a difference in one of the patients' lives, his secret is not to give up, to always persevere. He learned this technique early in his life, when he suffered his first bout with sickle cell anemia as a child.

What is sickle cell disease?

Sickle cell disease is a disease of the blood, sometimes known as sickle cell anemia. Red blood cells, when seen under the microscope, are normally round. When you have sickle cell anemia, many of your cells will have a different shape—that of a crescent moon, or a farmer's sickle. These odd-shaped cells are called sickle cells, and the disease they cause is sickle cell anemia.

Red blood cells carry hemoglobin molecules, which transport oxygen from your lungs throughout your body.

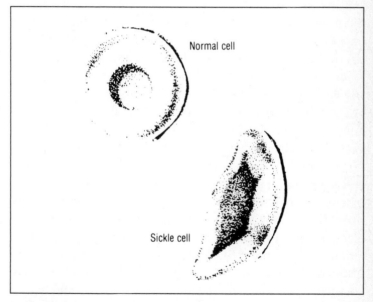

FIGURE 7A

Normal and sickle cell.
Reprinted with permission of the March of Dimes, from *Public Health Information Sheet, Genetic Series, Sickle Cell Anemia.*

If you have the sickle cell disease, your hemoglobin molecules stick together after they release the oxygen. This sticking together, combined with the loss of oxygen, causes your hemoglobin molecules to form into long, rigid rods inside your red blood cells.

In relation to the sickle cell hemoglobin, you can be affected in one of two ways. You can either be "trait carrying," or you can actually have the disease. If you're "trait carrying," you don't have the symptoms of sickle cell disease (mentioned later in this chapter), but you can pass the trait on to your children, just as one of your parents passed the sickle cell trait to you. For example, civil rights leader Jesse Jackson carries the trait for sickle cell disease but is, obviously, very healthy. If you have the disease, on the other hand, you will most likely experience all the symptoms we'll discuss later in this chapter, and may need regular medical care as a result.

As we mentioned, if you have the disease, the lengthening of your hemoglobin causes your normally round-shaped red blood cells to take on the shape of a sickle. Also, your red blood cells can lose their flexibility, which makes it more difficult for them to pass through small blood vessels. These "sickle" shaped cells, which are now odd-shaped and sticky, can clog your small blood vessels, causing your healthy red blood cells to become stuck behind them. Whatever organ or tissue that this now-clogged vessel leads to is deprived of an adequate blood supply. This type of blockage is what causes most of the problems and pain that accompany sickle cell disease. Also, the life span of red blood cells, when sickled, is shortened to 10 to 20 days, whereas normal cells live about 120 days. This means that bone marrow can't make cells quickly enough, resulting in profound anemia (low red blood cell count).

There are two myths that surround sickle cell disease. One is that it is contagious. The truth is you cannot catch sickle cell disease from another person. A second myth is that people with the disease do not live past the age of 20. This, too, is untrue. There are may people with sickle cell disease who have lived to enjoy old age. In severe cases, death may come in childhood or early adulthood.

How do I know if I am a candidate for sickle cell disease?

Sickle cell disease is, as we mentioned, an inherited disease. It works like this: If both of your parents are trait carriers, and both parents passed a sickle cell hemoglobin gene on to you, then up to 49 percent of your red blood cells may have sickle cell hemoglobin. The rest of the hemoglobin in your red blood cells will be normal. If your parents passed the gene for sickle cell disease to you, it can have many different implications for your children.

1. If you carry the sickle cell trait (SA), and your partner has normal hemoglobin (AA), you have a 50 percent chance of conceiving a child with normal hemoglobin (AA), and a 50 percent chance of having a child who carries the sickle cell trait (SA). There is no chance that any of your children will actually have the disease.

2. If you have sickle cell disease (SS) and your partner has normal hemoglobin (AA), all the children you conceive will carry the sickle cell trait (SA). None of your children will be born with normal hemoglobin (AA). But the good news is, none of your children will actually have the sickle cell disease (SS).

3. If both you and your partner carry the sickle cell trait (SA), you have a 25 percent chance of having a child

with normal hemoglobin (AA); a 50 percent chance of conceiving a child who carries the sickle cell trait (SA); and a 25 percent chance of having a child with sickle cell disease (SS).

4. If you carry the trait for sickle cells (SA) and your partner has the disease (SS), you have a 50 percent chance of having a child who carries the trait (SA), and a 50 percent chance of conceiving a child with sickle cell disease (SS).

5. If both you and your partner have sickle cell disease (SS), all your children will have the disease as well (SS).

6. If neither you nor your partner carries the trait or has the disease (AA), there is no chance that any of your children will have sickle cell disease.

Years ago, if both partners carried the trait for sickle cell disease, or had the disease, it was common for a doctor to discourage such a couple from having children. Today, doctors will generally make parents-to-be aware of the complications that their child may encounter. But whether or not the couple chooses to have a child is ultimately up to them.

What are the symptoms and signs of sickle cell disease?

The primary symptom of sickle cell disease is pain brought on by a sickle cell crisis, or a blockage in a blood vessel. If you have the disease, you may feel pain anywhere in your body and at any time. The intensity and frequency of these episodes vary with each person. Fletcher, for example, averages one or two incidents of pain each year; you may have more or less frequent occurrences. The intensity of your pain may also vary. Sometimes, if you have sickle cell disease, the pain can be so intense that you need to be hospitalized. This is only necessary until your pain subsides and the crisis in your blood is resolved.

Anemia

Anemia (hence the name sickle cell "anemia") is a common consequence of the disease. Anemia simply means that you have a low blood count or a decrease in your normal level of red blood cells. The sickled cell has a greatly shortened life span (two weeks), compared to the life span of a normal healthy red blood cell (about 120 days).

Bone marrow, which produces your red blood cells, can't keep up with the short life span of your sickled cells. If you have anemia, you may experience a headache, weakness, dizziness, perhaps nausea, and your skin may appear pale in color.

Jaundice

Another symptom of sickle cell disease is jaundice, when the white part of your eye turns yellowish. Called *icteric sclera,* this condition is usually not painful and may be a sign that blood cells are breaking up within your blood vessels.

Aseptic necrosis

Aseptic necrosis is the name given to deterioration and loss of bone, secondary to lost or poor blood supply to that area. This condition can often be confused with arthritis; however, the pain is usually more severe.

Leg ulcers

If you have sickle cell disease, ulcers may form around your ankles because of poor circulation. So if you have been diagnosed with sickle cell disease, pay attention to any sores that seem to be slow in healing, or chronic swelling of your thighs, and show these physical changes to your doctor for advice on early treatment.

Priapism

Common in young males, priapism occurs when a painful erection is experienced because of two cells sickling in the penis. Episodes like this can be caused by prolonged intercourse, masturbation or infection. Warm baths and immediate emptying of your bladder may reduce the discomfort or lessen the problem; however, if priapism persists for longer than 3 hours, seek medical attention for pharmacological intervention.

Sickle cell disease and blacks

One in every ten black Americans carries the sickle cell trait, and an estimated one out of every 400 black babies is born in the United States each year with sickle cell disease. Although the disorder affects more blacks than people of other races, some individuals who originate from the Caribbean, Latin America, the Mediterranean, Middle Eastern areas and Southeast Asia or India also suffer from the disease. Fifty thousand Americans have sickle cell disease, making it a significant health problem in the U.S. today.[1] Sickle cell disease cannot, as yet, be cured, but the symptoms can be made less severe with drugs and surgery.

Some experts say that the prevalence of sickle cell disease among blacks is due to our African roots. Ironically, it's a survival-of-the-fittest story. If you have sickle cell trait, you are protected against the deadly disease of malaria because malaria can attack only healthy cells. If you were born with sickle cells in a country ravaged by malaria, such as Africa or Haiti, you had a greater chance of survival than many of those around you without the sickle cell trait. As a result, in these countries, those with the sickle cell trait survived and grew up to have children who inherited the sickle cell trait. When their children moved away to other areas of the world, they took the disease with them and continued to pass it to future generations.

Fletcher copes with pain

Sometimes Fletcher's pain gets bad. Since he was born, he's had pain in every part of his body, depending on where his sickled cells decide to clog. He's lucky, though, because he gets the bad pain only once or twice a year. Other people with sickle cell anemia aren't as lucky, because they don't practice as many prevention techniques as Fletcher. Fletcher learned when he was very young how to prevent his pains from happening. He takes good care of himself and tries to avoid developing infections, a difficult feat considering that he works at a hospital and spends most of his time visiting people who are not well.

Usually, Fletcher fends off serious infections by asking his doctor to prescribe antibiotics at their early onset.

But every once in a while, one will develop that sends his body into a tailspin. If his pain is too bad, Fletcher is admitted to the hospital, where he receives treatment and pain medication until the crisis resolves. It usually takes a few days; then Fletcher is back at work, without much more than a memory of the earlier pain. He's lucky, and he knows it.

When Fletcher is admitted to the hospital, he usually meets other people with sickle cell anemia, many of whom are there for the fifth, sixth, even the tenth time that year. Fletcher has learned that he is very fortunate because his disease is less severe than that of most sickle cell patients. Part of the reason for this is that he takes very good care of himself and avoids dehydration and exposure to extreme temperatures, both factors that can lead to a sickle cell crisis.

Fletcher has learned that many of the other sickle cell patients he meets don't take as much care as he does to avoid painful crises. He always talks to them, asks how they are, and, before they know it, he's telling them how they can avoid infection and prevent unnecessary and uncomfortable hospital stays. They can't help but listen. Fletcher is not one who gives up easily.

How to avoid infection

Here are some of the tips that Fletcher usually shares with his newfound friends. Some of these can be very difficult to accomplish all the time, but it's helpful to be aware of what may be leading to your crises.

1. Try to stay clear of people with certain contagious infections; for example: flu, strep throat, etc.
2. With early signs of infection such as a cough, pain during urination, sore throat or fever, see your doctor

immediately. Have a culture taken and ask to be treated with antibiotics, if appropriate. Also, rest, drink lots of fluids and ask your doctor about other medications that may help you to recover quickly.

3. If you develop a sore, abrasion or cut on your skin, make sure you seek medical treatment immediately. Ask your physician about topical or oral antibiotics you can use to prevent any infection from spreading, and keep the affected area clean.

4. If you develop infected cysts or pus pockets, these usually need to be drained. Antibiotics alone may not do the job of clearing such infections.

5. Take preventive measures, such as getting flu shots or immunizations or taking preventive medications when traveling to certain countries. The health department is a good resource for information about these measures. Of course, consult your doctor before taking any medication or vaccines.

6. Avoid extreme temperatures.

7. Avoid caffeine and alcohol, and drink plenty of water every day, to limit your chances of becoming dehydrated.

What complications can I experience?

Not everyone with sickle cell disease will have all the symptoms and complications we've discussed. One sickle cell patient may have a few complications, while another may have an entirely different experience with the disease. A percentage of sickle cell patients may experience all of those mentioned.

Most of the complications of sickle cell disease are caused by sickling of your red blood cells, which partially or fully prevents oxygenated blood from reaching your organs. If an artery leading to one of your vital organs is blocked by sickled cells for a long period of time, it can cause irreparable damage. While pain resulting from the blockage can be lessened through narcotics, no one has yet discovered any method of preventing the sickling from happening in the first place. The area where the sickling occurs is very important because a blockage in an artery leading to certain areas, such as your brain, can be life-threatening. It can also be dangerous to have sickling for an extended period in vital organs such as your heart, liver, kidney, lungs or eyes.

Damage to your eyes due to clotting is one serious problem caused by sickle cell disease. Many people with the disease will appear to have yellow eyes, due to the breakdown of red blood cells. Your retina, the part of your eye that provides your brain with the information about what your eye is seeing, is especially sensitive to oxygen and blood loss. If clotting in your retina lasts for a long period of time, it can irreparably damage your vision.

Another problem is that the complications that are associated with sickle cell disease can easily be confused with the symptoms of other diseases or problems. Life-threatening diseases can be misdiagnosed as sickle cell disease, or vice versa. If you know you have sickle cell disease, be sure to tell your doctor so that he or she will not confuse the symptoms of sickle cell disease with other illnesses.

Should I be tested for sickle cell disease?

Even if you have never experienced any of the symptoms that we described earlier, as a member of a high-risk minority, you should still be tested for the sickle cell disease. The test that will show you if you have the disease, hemoglobin electrophoresis, is uncomplicated and can easily be arranged by your doctor or any health care professional. Hemoglobin electrophoresis will also show if you carry the sickle cell trait. This will be valuable information to you and your partner, when planning your family. It's a good idea for your whole family to be tested for the sickle cell trait.

Treating the disease

As yet, there is no cure for sickle cell disease. Complications of the disease can usually be treated with drugs, surgery, antibiotics, pain medication or simple bed rest. Prevention is important. Like Fletcher, you can lessen the number of episodes you have by taking good care of yourself. Try to avoid infections of all kinds, because any infection can lead to a sickle cell episode. Exercise regularly, but not too strenuously. Eat a proper diet and drink an excess amount of water (at least eight glasses) every day. Extra fluids can help your body ward off a sickle cell crisis. Finally, get enough rest and try to avoid stress whenever possible. (See Chapter Two for more information about how to prevent general diseases and infections.)

Conclusion

If you have sickle cell disease, take the time to learn about your disease and how best to cope with its complications. Follow the guidelines outlined in this book, use common sense and listen to what your body is telling you. By following these simple tips, like Fletcher, you too can benefit from a healthier life.

Resources

National Association for Sickle Cell Disease
3345 Wilshire Blvd., Suite 1106
Los Angeles, CA 90010-1880
(800) 421-8453
(203) 736-5455 (in California)

(The Association will provide you with genetic counseling and brochures; they will refer you to an office in your area for more information and possible financial aid.)

National Heart, Lung, and Blood Institute
Information Center
PO Box 30105
Bethesda, MD 20824-0105
(301) 951-3260

◆

8

Kidney Disease

Marcus's Story

Marcus is 58 years old. He and his wife own four dry-cleaning stores, which employ 50 people. Marcus has been working his way up the economic ladder ever since he quit school at the age of 14 to work at a dry cleaner's to help support his family. By the time he turned 20 years old, he was managing a cleaning store. As manager, he saved his money wisely until he could afford to start his own business. His business was such a success he added three more stores to his chain within a period of eight years.

Marcus is a hard worker and a smooth talker. He also has kidney disease. Since the age of 45 Marcus has had to receive dialysis therapy (the use of an artificial kidney to provide the same functions as the kidney) because his *disease has resulted in kidney failure. Marcus had some difficulty adapting to dialysis. Three days a week he spends several hours on dialysis in a renal clinic. He gets restless and fidgety, worrying about his four dry-cleaning stores. His wife, however, always assures him the business is fine, being run by his sons while he is gone.*

What is kidney disease?

Kidney disease is, basically, any disorder that causes dysfunction of your kidneys. There are many different types of kidney disease that stem from a variety of causes. Unfortunately, some of these causes are not yet fully understood. What is known is that any disease of your kidney usually affects both kidneys, and if the damage is serious enough, kidney failure, also called end state renal disease (ESRD), will occur.

In order to better understand what kidney disease (also known as renal disease) is, it is important to understand the functions of the kidneys. Approximately 400 gallons of blood flow through your kidneys each day via your renal artery, which connects your kidneys directly to your body's main blood vessel, the aorta. Blood enters your kidneys and passes through nephrons, which act as tiny filters. Many substances sent through your kidneys are reabsorbed into your bloodstream. Wastes that are filtered out of the blood are sent through your ureters (one tube is attached to each kidney) and then on to your bladder, where they are stored until released from the body through your urethra as urine.

Your kidneys have many functions, in addition to making urine or waste removal. These include balancing the chemicals in your body (for example, sodium and potassium), balancing certain hormones (such as renin), and

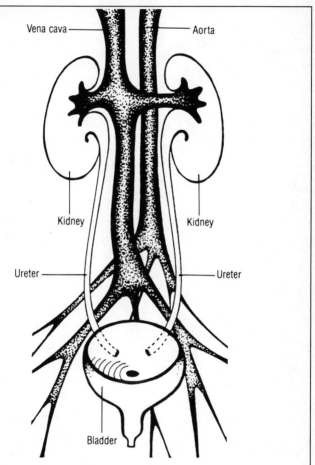

The kidneys are located behind your other abdominal organs. The vessels that connect them with the circulatory system are shown above. The large vessel at the right is the aorta; that at the left, the vena cava. Descending from the kidneys are the ureters, which empty into the bladder (at bottom of drawing).

FIGURE 8A

The kidneys, ureters, and bladder.
Reprinted with permission of the National Kidney Foundation, from "Your Kidneys: Master Chemists of the Body," 1984.

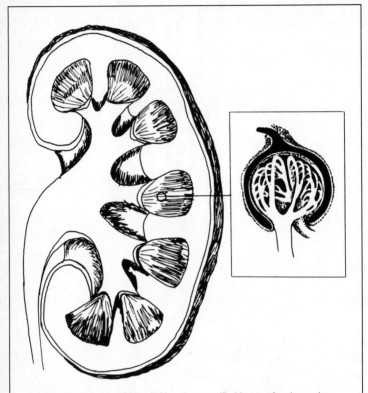

A cross section of a kidney (left) and a magnified image of a glomerulus. Glomeruli are the delicate structures that filter wastes from the blood.

FIGURE 8B

Cross section of a kidney.
Reprinted with permission of Diabetes Forecast, from "Kidney Treatment Today."

regulating your body fluids. The interesting thing about kidneys is that while two are certainly ideal, one is really all you need to adequately balance the waste and chemicals in your body.

Kidney disease and blacks

According to data released by the United States Renal Data System (USRDS) Annual Data Report 1990, ESRD (end stage renal disease) is more prevalent among blacks than whites. In 1988, there were 172,506 ESRD patients in the Medicare system, representing approximately 93 percent of all ESRD patients in the United States.[1] Of that number, 67 percent (115,014) were white, 4 percent (7,913) were other races, and 29 percent (49,579) were black.[2] Considering that blacks make up only 12 percent of the general American population, the number of blacks with ESRD is disproportionally high.

There are currently 150,000 patients nationwide in an ESRD program, a number that is projected to increase to 250,000 in the year 2000, according to the National Kidney Foundation, Inc.

What causes kidney disease?

There are many diseases associated with the kidney. All of these disorders and diseases can be classified in one of the following two categories: hereditary or congenital disorders, and acquired disorders.

Hereditary and congenital disease

Hereditary kidney diseases are just what they sound like—they're passed down through your family. Polycystic kidney disease, a disorder in which your kidneys are filled with small balloon-type spaces, is the most common form of hereditary kidney disease. We will explain this disorder more fully later in this chapter. Some congenital abnormalities are structural problems that you have inherited from your parents (for example, a narrow or missing part of your ureter). Congenital kidney disease occurs in utero and may or may not be inherited.

Acquired kidney disease

Acquired kidney disease is the most common form of kidney problem. Acquired diseases can begin from an infection, such as strep throat, and then lead to kidney damage. To prevent acquired diseases, it's important to take good care of yourself. Refer to Chapter Two for additional ways to prevent infections and minor disorders that can put you at greater risk for kidney complications.

Types of kidney disease

There are a wide variety of diseases starting primarily in the kidney, some of which can lead to total kidney failure. However, if caught in the early stages, many of these diseases can be effectively treated so that the kidney will still partially function. Following are some specific examples of common types of kidney diseases.

Kidney stones

No one knows why some people are more prone to kidney stones than others. What is known is that approximately 200,000 people in the United States are admitted to the hospital each year because of pain and complications due to kidney stones. This figure includes only those patients whose kidney stone problems were serious

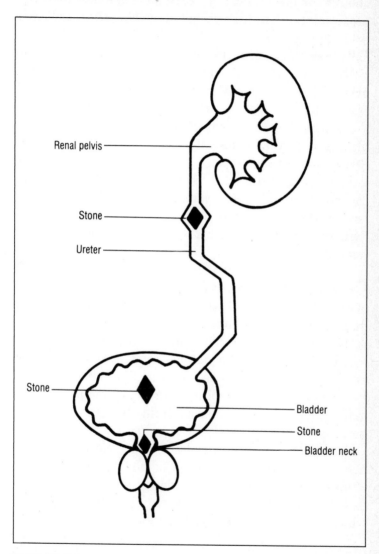

FIGURE 8C

Kidney stone.
Reprinted with permission of the National Kidney Foundation, from "About Kidney Stones," 1988.

enough for hospitalization. Estimates are that up to approximately 1.5 million people in the United States suffer from kidney stones.

Kidney stones are caused by the mineral composition of the urine, which favors formations of stones. Over a period of time, certain minerals build up to form hard stones of various shapes and sizes. Problems occur when the stones lodge in areas of your kidney or ureters to block the flow of urine, thus causing kidney damage. Stones can also cause bleeding in your urine and may lead to urinary infections. Some stones are so small they can pass through your system without too many problems. Others, however, can get large enough to make them difficult or impossible to pass and cause excruciating pain.

Treatment for stones will differ with each person, depending on the composition and size of the stone. Only about 10 percent of all people with kidney stones have to undergo surgery to have them removed. Generally, the doctor will tell you to drink lots of fluids every day as a means of treating kidney stones, and as an easy way to prevent kidney stones from forming. By drinking lots of fluids, you continually dilute your urine and prevent too many concentrated minerals from depositing in your kidneys.

Your doctor may also prescribe medication that can help to prevent the formation of new stones. Another, more recent development in kidney stone treatment is called extracorporeal shock-wave lithostripy (ESWL), which breaks up stones by shock waves.

Glomerulonephritis

Glomeruli are intertwined masses of thin-walled capillaries (blood vessels) where filtration takes place in your kidneys. Glomerulonephritis occurs when these capillaries become inflamed or destroyed. When these capillaries are damaged, your internal filtering system becomes less efficient, allowing more protein and blood to enter your urine. There are two types of glomerulonephritis: acute and chronic.

Acute glomerulonephritis occurs primarily in children and is often discovered when blood is seen in the urine. Other symptoms include puffiness in your face and increased blood pressure. This type of kidney disease may clear up by itself, but the high blood pressure that accompanies the disorder can cause serious problems.

Chronic glomerulonephritis means you have a continual or persistent kidney problem. Unlike acute glomerulonephritis, the chronic version develops slowly and usually causes much more permanent damage to your kidneys than acute. To find out if you have chronic glomerulonephritis, look for frequent urination, bloody or dark-colored urine, a puffy face and high blood pressure. While these symptoms do not always mean you have this condition, they should be taken seriously. If you are experiencing these symptoms, seek medical help immediately. Chronic glomerulonephritis may not result in total kidney failure but you may require kidney dialysis. You may improve your condition by changing your diet to foods that are low in salt and protein. Your doctor can also explain other treatments to you, depending on the type of glomerulonephritis and symptoms you have.

Polycystic kidney disease

Another kidney disease, polycystic kidney disease, is characterized by the formation of cysts or small balloon-type pockets in your kidney. This condition is hereditary. While there is currently no cure, if you have this disease, it is important to seek treatment early. It may be a good idea to ask your relatives if there is any history of kidney disease in your family. If there is, look for potential symptoms and signs such as lower back pain (caused by the cysts), recurrent urinary infections and bleeding and high blood pressure. If you suspect kidney trouble, seek medical help immediately.

Nephrosis

If your kidneys filter too much protein from your blood into your urine, there's a good chance you have nephrosis. This loss of protein causes fluid to leak into your body's tissues, leading to salt and fluid retention that causes puffiness (edema) in areas such as your eyes, feet and face. This condition can lead to kidney failure. However, if you have nephrosis, you'll be happy to know that it has been known to disappear spontaneously. In some cases, nephrosis patients can also be effectively treated with drugs, such as steroids.

Pyelonephritis

Sometimes urine can back up from your bladder into one of your kidneys, because of a faulty door or valve found between your bladder and ureter. When this happens, the bacteria in your urine can infect your kidneys, causing a condition called pyelonephritis.

If you experience a burning sensation when urinating, frequent urination, chills, fever or blood in your urine, you may have this condition. If you suspect you're at risk, seek medical help immediately, since you can be cured of pyelonephritis with antibiotics. If left untreated, it can lead to end stage renal disease (kidney failure).

Diabetes

Diabetes is the most common cause of ESRD. Between 1986 and 1988, diabetes caused 32.2 percent of new ESRD cases. When you suffer from Type II (adult onset) diabetes, you have approximately a 10 percent chance of experiencing severe kidney failure. When the blood vessels in your kidneys are injured, your kidneys cannot clean your blood properly. Injury will probably be first detected with the discovery of protein in your urine by routine laboratory tests. When the level of protein in your blood drops with an increase in protein in your urine, you'll probably experience swelling in your ankles and legs, and puffiness in your face. These changes may cause you to use the bathroom more at night and may cause your blood pressure to rise.

As your kidney fails, other changes will also be detected in your laboratory blood tests. You may experience nausea, vomiting, a loss of appetite, weakness, increasing tiredness, itching, muscle cramps (especially in your legs) and anemia (a low blood count).

Keeping good control of your diabetes will lower your risk of having severe kidney disease. You need to get eight hours of sleep, follow your diabetic diet, take medications or insulin as indicated, and you must get regular exercise. It's also important to avoid alcohol and cigarettes. (See Chapter Five for more information on diabetes.)

High blood pressure

According to the Bureau of Health Statistics, 27 percent of all renal failure cases may be caused by high blood pressure.[3] Therefore, by controlling your high blood pressure with medicine and other preventive measures (see Chapter Three), your chance of preventing kidney failure is very good. High blood pressure damages your kidneys' blood vessels, causing them to become thick and rigid. This, in turn reduces the blood supply to your kidneys. Then your kidneys can't remove waste products, which can result in your body's slowly becoming poisoned. Dialysis or a kidney transplant is then necessary.

Uremia

If your kidneys have failed and you become anemic (a direct result of ESRD), you probably have a condition called uremia. Since your kidneys are no longer functioning properly—they're not filtering wastes or toxins from your blood—these wastes (urea is one example) build up in your blood, slowly poisoning your body. You may experience many different reactions as a result of uremic syndrome:

- When your kidneys are not functioning properly, they are no longer able to filter *potassium* from your blood. As mentioned earlier, too much potassium in your body can lead to an irregular heartbeat and can affect your muscle function.
- Healthy kidneys release the hormone *erythropoietin* into your blood, which stimulates red blood cell production. If you have uremia, your erythropoietin levels decrease, slowing down red blood cell production and causing you to become anemic. If you are experiencing pale skin, fatigue and low energy levels, you may be anemic.
- When your kidneys fail, they no longer filter and balance *sodium* levels in your body. As a result, high levels of sodium build up, causing you to retain

water and causing the volume of blood within your
blood vessels to increase. These increased fluid levels
cause high blood pressure.

◆ If you have uremia, you may also notice that your
skin has become *yellowish* in color. This phenomenon
is caused by urinary pigment building up in your
blood.

◆ If your kidneys are damaged, they do not release
the proper amount of vitamin D, which aids in the
absorption of calcium by the bones; this can cause
your *bones* to weaken. Instead of storing calcium,
your bones release it, causing calcium buildup in
your soft tissues.

◆ Your *nervous system* can be sedated in the final
stages of uremia, resulting in a coma, unless dialysis
or transplant is implemented.

Kidney failure

There are two types of kidney failure: ESRD (end stage
renal disease) and acute kidney failure. In acute kidney
failure, your disease may clear up with a change in diet,
regulation of fluids and administration of certain medications. Dialysis is seldom needed. ESRD, on the other
hand, is usually not reversible.

Acute kidney failure

Acute kidney failure sometimes occurs after you experience a severe infection, some type of trauma (such
as sudden loss of blood or significant lowering of blood
pressure), poisoning, an accident or burn. Sometimes, the
cause of your kidney failure might be unknown. In other
cases, a blockage in the blood vessels leading to your
kidneys, an incompatible blood transfusion, or certain

kidney diseases may lead to your disorder. Once treated, your kidneys may resume functioning normally after a few days to several weeks.

To detect acute kidney failure, look for a decrease of urine output, swelling and high blood pressure.

End stage renal disease (ESRD)

ESRD means your kidneys are not capable of working hard enough to keep you alive. In other words, treatment is essential to help your kidneys do their job. ESRD can be caused by many diseases, but in blacks it is usually the result of diabetes or high blood pressure (hypertension), especially among young black men. If you are at risk for high blood pressure, the single most important thing you can do to prevent kidney failure is to keep your blood pressure in check. (See Chapter Three for ways to do this.) If your chronic renal disease has caused your kidneys to lose 90 to 95 percent of their functioning ability, there are only two ways a medical professional can keep you alive—dialysis or a kidney transplant. Unlike in acute kidney failure, in ESRD your kidneys usually do not regain their ability to function.

As you have probably realized after reading the chapters on high blood pressure and diabetes, all of these diseases are interrelated. Approximately 27 percent of all ESRD cases are caused by hypertension and 32 percent are caused by diabetes.[4] Keeping your blood pressure and diabetes under control are important strategies when it comes to preventing ESRD.

How do I know if I have kidney disease?

If you have kidney disease, the cleaning process of your blood will not be affected until two-thirds of your total kidney mass is affected. During this time you may not know you are sick because the early stages of kidney disease have no symptoms. Fortunately, urine and blood tests can be used to detect early signs of kidney disease.

Urine tests

For years, dating back to Hippocrates, physicians have known enough about urine to know that it can very often hold the answer to a diagnosis. In ancient times, physicians used to taste urine in order to detect diabetes mellitus. The urine of a diabetic contains excess sugar (glucose), so it should taste sweet. When your kidneys are damaged, as we've stated earlier, the filtering process is no longer working properly. As a result, there will be an excess of certain substances in your urine.

It's no wonder, then, that your doctor may usually request a urine sample during your checkup. Besides indicating a kidney disorder, a urinalysis can indicate a problem somewhere else in your body.

Following are some of the things your physician or medical professional looks for in a urinalysis.

- In healthy patients, only trace amounts of protein can be found in urine samples. On the other hand, if you have kidney disease, an increased amount of protein can often be detected (proteinuria).
- An excess of glucose in your urine can be a sign of diabetes, kidney disease, or both.
- Bacteria in the urine is a sign of kidney or bladder infection.
- Too much or too little acid content in your urine may also indicate kidney disease.
- Blood or pus in your urine is another indication of kidney disease.

The nitrite test

You can also test your urine for infection at home. Nitrite urine testing kits can be bought at a pharmacy. They contain special chemically treated paper strips, which are to be inserted into an early morning urine sample. The color of the strip will change if bacteria-producing nitrite is present. This test tends to be about 70 percent accurate.

Blood tests

Often, you will be given a blood test in combination with a urine test. Too many waste products in your blood indicate that your kidneys are not doing their job properly. There may be elevations of the substance blood urea nitrogen (BUN), or creatinine (Creat).

Cystoscopy

A cystoscopy is a procedure in which your doctor uses an instrument to look into your bladder. The instrument used, a cytoscope, is lighted and has attachments that can lift out small stones found in your bladder or ureters, burn off tumors, and clear obstructions.

X rays and other procedures

X rays of the kidney can be taken with or without dye. When dye is used, it is injected into a vein and is eventually filtered through the kidneys. By taking X rays every few minutes, doctors can see how the dye collects in your kidney, ureters, and bladder.

There are also more sophisticated tests using computerized X rays and radioactive isotopes.

Marcus perseveres

Marcus, the dry-cleaning entrepreneur, says he felt like he was wasting a lot of hours during dialysis that could have been spent at the stores. One day, his sons pointed out that he could get a lot of work done during dialysis. Today, Marcus takes all the accounting books, order forms, and a cellular phone so that he can do business during dialysis. He balances the books, places orders, and handles customer and personnel problems all from the dialysis center. Quick with a sales pitch and his business card, Marcus also drums up new business from nurses, doctors and patients alike.

Treatment of end stage renal disease

As recently as in the 1950s, ESRD was considered a fatal condition. The medical community has made great strides in treating this disease since then. If you acquire ESRD, you have three major treatment options: hemodialysis, peritoneal dialysis and kidney transplantation.

Hemodialysis

Hemodialysis is a process by which toxins, minerals and fluids are removed from your body by circulating your blood through an artificial kidney called a dialyzer. Basically, this machine does what your kidneys should be doing, filtering your blood. Instead of using nephrons, capillaries and membranes to do the job, a hemodialysis machine uses a special filter or dialyzer.

During hemodialysis, blood is taken through tubes to the dialyzer, which takes out wastes and excess fluids. The filtered blood then goes back through another set of tubes into your body. Hemodialysis must usually be

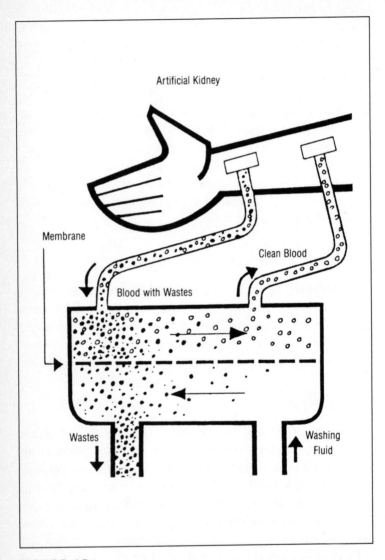

FIGURE 8D

Hemodialysis.
Reprinted with permission of the National Kidney Foundation, "Dialysis," 1991.

performed three times a week, and one session can last three to four hours. Some people prefer to receive treatment at home, with the help of a trained friend or family member. Others receive treatment at a hemodialysis center or clinic. During treatment, you may experience side effects, such as muscle cramps or a sudden drop in blood pressure. At times, you may feel weak and dizzy, because of the sudden change in body fluids and chemicals in your body. More serious side effects, such as nausea, vomiting and seizures, may also occur. Report all side effects to your doctor.

While on hemodialysis, you must adhere to a special diet, according to the U.S. Department of Health and Human Resources. Try to follow these guidelines:

◆ If we didn't have as much animal protein in our diet, it's suggested that there wouldn't be as many cases of kidney disease in the U.S. Reduce the amount of meat proteins you eat. If you do eat meat, try to eat fish and chicken. These contain adequate quantities of protein to maintain muscle normality.

◆ Be cautious about the amount of potassium you consume. Too much or too little potassium can be harmful.

◆ Be very careful about how much liquid you drink. Too much liquid gives your kidneys much more to do and will make your tissues swell in addition to causing high blood pressure and heart trouble.

◆ Stay away from salt. Salt attracts water, and too much water can cause problems in patients with kidney failure. The combination of excess salt and water will result in swelling.

◆ Limit foods such as milk, cheese, nuts, dried beans and soft drinks, since they contain high amounts of phosphorus. Phosphorus can cause calcium to be extracted from your bones, weakening them.

Peritoneal dialysis

Peritoneal Dialysis (PD) is an alternative dialytic therapy that uses part of your own body—the lining of your abdominal cavity, the peritoneal membrane—to filter your blood. This is done by placing a catheter and a sterile cleansing solution, called dialysate, into your abdominal cavity. The dialysis catheter is placed in an area below your navel and remains there throughout dialysis. All the wastes, excess fluid and chemicals pass into the dialysate from blood vessels in your peritoneal membrane. The dialysate is drained from your body after several hours, at which time fresh dialysate is introduced and the whole process begins again.

There are three types of peritoneal dialysis:

1. *Continuous Ambulatory Peritoneal Dialysis (CAPD)* is the type of dialysis most used by people suffering from end stage renal disease. The term "ambulatory" comes from the fact that the dialysis can take place while you are moving about during the day. No machine is used with this type of dialysis. The dialysate enters the catheter in your abdomen from a plastic bag. With the catheter sealed, the dialysate remains in your abdomen for four to six hours, and then the dialysate is drained from your abdomen back into the bag. Fresh dialysate is then added and the process begins again. The bag can be hidden under your clothes, so those around you do not even have to know that you're undergoing dialysis. One positive aspect of CAPD is that the treatment can be taken care of

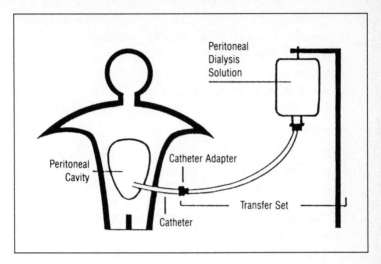

FIGURE 8E

Peritoneal dialysis.
Reprinted with permission of the National Kidney Foundation, "Dialysis," 1991.

entirely by the patient—you don't need a machine or professional assistance. Perhaps the most unpopular aspect of this type of treatment is that you have to carry the bag around all day. If you use this type of dialysis, you'll usually have to change the dialysate four times a day.

2. *Continuous Cyclic Peritoneal Dialysis (CCPD)* is just like CAPD, except the treatments take place while you sleep. A machine automatically fills and drains the solution to and from your abdominal cavity. Unlike CAPD, you must use a machine and you need assistance from another person. Treatments take approximately 10 to 12 hours and must be done every day.

3. *Intermittent Peritoneal Dialysis (IPD)* is a longer treatment process than CCPD; however, the same type of machine is used to exchange dialysate. Generally, this type of treatment occurs at the hospital, but it can also be performed at home. IPD must be done several times a week, for a weekly total of 36 to 42 hours.

According to the U.S. Department of Health and Human Services, your diet for peritoneal dialysis is slightly different from that for hemodialysis:

- You may be able to have more salt and fluids.
- You should eat more protein.
- You may need to cut back on the number of calories you consume, because sugar in the dialysate can cause you to gain weight.

Kidney transplantation

Gary Coleman, the former star of the hit television show *Diff'rent Strokes,* has had kidney disease all his life. Despite his affliction, Coleman has maintained an active career as a television and screen star. He is also the recipient of many sequential kidney transplants.

Fifty-eight percent of all patients on the transplant waiting list are black. In 1989, black organ donors represented 15 percent of total donors; in 1990, black organ donors represented 8 percent of total donors. As of November 26, 1990, LIFELINK (a nonprofit organ tissue recovery center) reported 330 blacks awaiting a kidney transplant. Only seven of 84 donors that year were black.[5] Unfortunately, blacks tend to donate fewer kidneys than others. The likelihood of compatibility is greater if a black gets a kidney from a black cadaver or living donor. The number of black organ donors is dismal compared to the number of blacks waiting for kidneys. From these statistics, it is obvious that we need a stronger donor program.

In many instances, organ transplantation is the best option for people afflicted with this disease. Transplants can be obtained from living related donors or from cadavers. In other words, when a person dies with normal kidneys, for example, from an auto accident, if the victim's family notifies the emergency organ procurement program, they can donate their loved one's kidneys to help another person. Also, living relatives can donate one of their kidneys to a family member. The success rate with family donors is very high because your body is less likely to reject a kidney transplant from a body genetically similar to your own. The donor can live just fine with one kidney—that's really all we need.

If you are on dialysis and are interested in receiving a transplant, consult your doctor. He or she can advise you on how to begin the process of finding a suitable donor.

Conclusion

As you can see, your kidneys are critical to your health. Since many of the symptoms of kidney disease are not immediately visible and can cause serious damage to your body without your even knowing it, it's important to see your doctor regularly for checkups. A simple urinalysis and blood test are all it takes to detect immediate problems. Just as with any disease or illness, your diet can play an important role, both in prevention (especially when it comes to properly managing diabetes and high blood pressure) and treatment. Follow the guidelines listed in this chapter.

If you are in need of treatment for end stage renal disease, carefully consider your options. Remember, dialysis and transplantation are not cures, just treatments. Think over your decision carefully. The right treatment often depends on your present lifestyle and health condition.

Resources

American Association of Kidney Patients
Suite LL1
1 Davis Boulevard
Tampa, FL 33606
(813) 251-0725

(The Association helps patients locate support groups. It also offers information and brochures about living a better life as a dialysis patient. The membership fee of $15 each year covers costs of providing you with magazines, books and pamphlets.)

American Kidney Fund
Suite 1010
6110 Executive Boulevard
Rockville, MD 20852
(800) 638-8299

(The Kidney Fund can help you find sources of financial assistance. The organization also offers brochures and pamphlets—the first copy of each is free of charge.)

National Kidney Foundation, Inc.
30 East 33rd Street, 11th Floor
New York, NY 10016
(800) 622-9010

(The Foundation offers brochures and pamphlets on diet, blood pressure and general kidney disease treatments. All information is provided free. Your local Kidney Foundation organization can refer you to a support group.)

National Kidney and Urologic Diseases
   Information Clearinghouse
Box NKUDIC
9000 Rockville Pike
Bethesda, MD 20892
(301) 645-4415

(The Clearinghouse offers patient education information. They will do a free computer search for you on a comprehensive health database that provides bibliographies on kidney disease, audiovisual materials and fact sheets.)

AIDS and Sexually Transmitted Diseases

Jason's story

Even at the advanced stage of his illness, Jason didn't want anyone to know. His own mother was kept in the dark. She told everyone the same thing he told her— "He just couldn't get rid of his cold, he suspected he was anemic, and, yes, he had lost a great deal of weight, but there was this terrific new diet . . . " Jason is a young black man in his twenties, and he has AIDS.

A devoted athlete, Jason always took his body and its well-being seriously. Two years ago, he started noticing changes in his health. It seemed like he was sick with some sort of cold or flu all the time. Each time he got sick, it seemed to take him longer and longer to bounce back. Before he started getting sick, Jason would run every morning before work. About a year ago, however, he began sleeping in more often, never quite finding the energy to get up, pull on his shoes and shorts, and go running.

Jason even began to lose interest in bar-hopping and socializing with friends. He used to pride himself on being a ladies' man. He would go out several times a week to a variety of bars and mix and mingle. Sometimes, if he and one of the women he met really hit it off, they would go home together. After all, Jason was very liberal. Casual sex, in his opinion, was acceptable.

The sores were what finally convinced him to go to the doctor. They began to appear on his legs in small red circles. That frightened him. It also frightened the last woman he brought home.

Anyone can contract HIV, and there are a number of ways to catch the virus. Arthur Ashe, a famous black tennis star, contracted HIV through a blood transfusion. He had kept his illness private for years before finally admitting it to the public, then he spent the final ten months of his life teaching others about the disease before dying from AIDS in February 1993. Ervin "Magic" Johnson, a high-profile basketball player, formerly with the Los Angeles Lakers, is infected with HIV. He, too, has gone public with his HIV status and is trying to educate people about the disease.

What is HIV/AIDS?

AIDS (acquired immune deficiency syndrome) is a disease in which your body's immune system breaks down. Normally, your immune system fights off infections and diseases. But if you have AIDS your immune system fails, putting you at great risk of contracting life-threatening illnesses including severe pneumonia, cancer, and nervous system infections. Having AIDS is like being sent to war with no armor or ammunition—you're vulnerable to attack and have no way to fight back.

The healthy immune system is constantly fighting many types of viruses. Some, like those that cause colds, are a mild challenge. Others, like the human immunodeficiency virus (HIV), the virus that causes AIDS, can practically destroy your immune system.

HIV, like any other virus, enters your body and immediately begins replicating itself, destroying cells in its wake (although studies have shown that HIV can remain inactive in your body for some time before beginning this replication process). Your body may initially put up a strong defense to HIV, and it can take many years before a substantial number of your cells become infected. Unlike a cold virus, which announces its arrival a few days later in the form of a sneeze or sniffle, HIV may not show symptoms in your body for months or even years.

Even if you're not yet showing symptoms of HIV, the virus can be detected with blood tests. According to the Centers for Disease Control (CDC), 99.8 percent of people infected with HIV will test positive for the virus within six months after infection. By the time you begin to experience AIDS symptoms, your condition may be life-threatening.

How can I prevent becoming infected with HIV?

The best thing about HIV/AIDS is that you don't have to have it. Sure, there are going to be those rare accidental HIV infections over which no one has control, such as yourself, because no one else is going to do it for you. No one else cares as much as you do—after all, it's *your* life that is at risk.

If you've been tested recently for HIV and the test turned out negative, you're halfway there. Make sure the person you're having sex with is also tested. There's always the chance that even though you and your partner have tested negative once, you may be in a "window period"—less than six months after infection—when the virus can't be detected. You must have two tests, six months apart, with no risky behavior in between, in order to be sure you're HIV negative. Unless you're completely sure, always wear a condom, and never, ever use a condom more than once.

Latex condoms protect you and your partner from each other's body fluids. The semen of an HIV-infected person will contain the virus and you want to make it impossible for HIV-infected semen to enter your or your partner's bloodstream.

Condoms are packaged very small and don't take up much room, so make it a practice to carry them with you at all times. Just don't store them in your glove compartment or wallet because heat can destroy the latex. Find a size that's right for you. A loose-fitting condom serves no purpose and will prove uncomfortable for you and your partner. Make sure you also check the expiration date—after a certain amount of time, condoms begin to lose their effectiveness.

How to use a condom

1. Remove the condom from the package carefully, looking for tears in the packaging. Do not handle the condom in a manner that may rip its latex. (For example,

when a nurse or a doctor is accidentally stuck wit
infected needle. The majority of AIDS cases, however
caused by unprotected sex or sharing needles when u
drugs. You can control these risks. By taking prec
tions, you could very well save your own life.

Use condoms

It's the Age of the Condom. Many years ago, condom
were introduced as a birth-control method. Today, th
condom is also used as protection from HIV and othe
sexually transmitted diseases. Not so long ago, it was
considered embarrassing to have to go to the drug store to
purchase them. Today, condoms are handed out on street
corners and college campuses and are even sold in their
own specialty stores. They now come in every color and
style imaginable, even glow-in-the-dark! No matter what
color, shape or design you prefer, be sure to use only condoms made of latex.

*Just remember—condoms are not 100 percent
safe in protecting against HIV. They can break or
slip off, or even have a hole in them.* Yet as imperfect
as condoms may be, they have become essential in fighting the war against HIV/AIDS. The only sure way to
avoid HIV/AIDS is to abstain from sex, avoid sharing
needles, or to have sex with only one mutually faithful
partner, who has repeatedly tested negative for HIV.

If you're not sure if you or your partner is infected with
HIV, always wear or have your partner wear a condom.
A condom should be used for sex, not just during the
act, but during foreplay and afterplay as well. A condom
should be used when you put your penis inside the mouth,
rectum or vagina of your partner. You should also use
condoms, whether your partner is male or female. Protect

1 PUTTING IT ON

- Use a new condom before each sex act.

- When penis is hard (before any sexual contact), place condom on tip and roll down all the way.

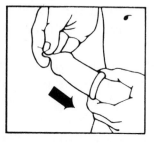

- Squeeze tip of condom to remove air. (Excess air could cause condom to break.)

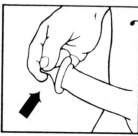

2 TAKING IT OFF

- After coming, withdraw penis while still hard.

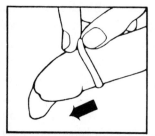

- Hold on to rim of condom as you withdraw so nothing spills.

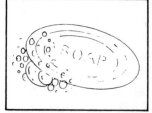

- Avoid further sexual contact with your partner until both of you wash your sex organs and any other areas that came in contact with body fluids.

FIGURE 9A

How to use a condom.
From the Ansell Medical Products booklet "How to Use a Condom" (Reprinted with permission).

don't use your teeth to rip open the package.) If anything appears at all wrong with the condom, discard it. Risking an unwanted pregnancy or HIV transmission is just not worth it.

2. With your thumb and finger, gently squeeze the tip of the condom. Make sure there will be room in the tip for your semen to collect. Then, place the rolled-up condom at the tip of your erect penis and roll down. Prevent any air pockets from forming. Roll the condom to the base of your penis.

3. One factor that causes problems with condom use is lack of lubrication. Dry friction can cause the condom to tear or break. Water-based lubricants, nonallergenic surgical lubricants (K-Y Jelly), and some contraceptive jellies and foams can be helpful. These products are available in pharmacies and sex specialty shops. Make sure you always read labels. **Do not use petroleum jelly or any oil-based lubricant such as hand or body lotion, skin moisturizer or food products because these will dissolve the condom's latex.** Also, do not use saliva, which may contain germs or blood. Contraceptive jelly, creams and foams contain nonoxynol-9, a chemical that destroys disease-causing germs (including HIV), in addition to killing sperm.

4. After ejaculation and while it is still erect, remove your penis from your partner's body or have your partner remove his penis from yours, holding the base of the condom so that its contents do not slip onto your partner. This is important, because the penis gets soft after ejaculation, which means the condom may loosen and slip.

5. After use, dispose of the condom carefully, so that the

semen does not spill out. Never reuse a condom or use the same condom for the various types of sexual intercourse. New, unused condoms should be used for anal, oral and vaginal penetration.[1]

Dental dams

Dental dams are a relatively new concept in safe sex. A dental dam is a square sheet of latex that can be placed over the vagina or anus during oral sex, preventing the exchange of body fluids. You can purchase dental dams at your local pharmacy. If you don't have a dental dam, a nonlubricated condom can be unrolled and cut to the right size.

How do I know if I have HIV?

There's no way to know for sure if you have HIV, without having an HIV antibody test. When the human immunodeficiency virus enters your bloodstream, your immune system produces special antibodies to fight it. An HIV test reveals the presence of HIV antibodies in your blood.

Some people are reluctant to have the HIV test taken because they don't want anyone to know they are being tested. They worry that if their test results turn out to be positive, others will know they have HIV. The solution is to have an anonymous HIV test. No one has to know your name. If you do test positive, it's important to consult a health care professional immediately, to talk about the care you will need. Although no cure for HIV or AIDS has been found yet, there are still many things you can do to slow the process of the disease and keep yourself feeling well for a long time.

Two types of HIV tests

There are two types of tests used to detect HIV. The first, called ELISA, which stands for "enzyme-linked immunoabsorbent assay," tests for HIV-related antibodies. This is a very sensitive test, 98% accurate, and is the one that the American Red Cross usually uses to test blood that has been donated. Unfortunately, with this test, small particles like proteins and non-HIV antibodies are sometimes mistaken for HIV antibodies and trigger a false positive result. To double-check for this mistake, a second type of test, called the western blot, is used.

The western blot test is more specific, but also more expensive. For this reason, the western blot is used only to confirm a positive ELISA test. In this test an experienced technician, rather than a machine, interprets the results.

Blood test accuracy

If your blood is tested by both the ELISA and the western blot tests, you can be fairly sure that the results you get are accurate. In rare instances, "false positives" and "false negatives" have been reported. A "false positive" result means that although the test results report you are infected with HIV, you are not. A "false negative" occurs when the test results say you are not infected with HIV, yet you actually have the virus. "False negatives" occur most often during the "window period." This is the period after you have been infected with HIV, but before your body has built up enough HIV antibodies to be detected by an ELISA test.

If you know that you have been exposed to HIV, get tested at regular intervals so that no mistake is made.

Test results, depending on which kind of test is used and where you are tested, usually take about a week to get back. If you have a high risk of being exposed to HIV, and your initial test was negative, you should have follow-up testing six weeks and six months after the suspect exposure. And make sure you avoid unsafe sex and drug use.

Where should I get tested?

You can have an HIV antibody test at most health clinics, local health departments, hospitals or doctors' offices. However, if you are tested at any one of these places, there's no guarantee that your results will be kept confidential. Some hospitals and doctors are required by law to report those people who test positive for HIV. If you want to be assured of confidentiality, go to a site that offers anonymous testing. Call the Centers for Disease Control National AIDS Hotline: 1-800-342-AIDS, for information on anonymous testing sites in your area, or call your state health department. Many state and county health departments provide these blood tests free of charge for people who can't afford the fee.

Treatment

Imagine yourself in this scenario: You decide to have an HIV test. After all, you may have done something in your past, before AIDS became a threat, that put you at risk. Days later, the results come back. You have tested positive for being infected with HIV. Now what? Fear, anger, frustration, helplessness—these are all natural reactions you may feel. You've seen movies and read stories about people with AIDS. But this time, it's you.

Don't lose hope! Research is going on every day to find a cure for AIDS. There are currently many prescription medicines that can help prevent and treat HIV-related infections, and slow down the virus as it attacks your immune system. New drugs are being tested all over the world and clinical drug trials can give you access to investigational therapies.

The stages of HIV

If you are infected with HIV, it's important to understand the changes that are going on in your body. A positive test for HIV doesn't necessarily mean you have AIDS. There are four stages your body can go through:

1. *Before HIV antibodies show up on a test:* You can be infected with HIV but not have enough antibodies to be detected by a test. This "window period" we've mentioned earlier can last for several weeks or months after infection.
2. *HIV positive, but showing no symptoms:* If you've been told that you are HIV positive, or if you suspect that you have been exposed to HIV, but have no symptoms, you may be particularly dangerous to others. Because you may not be aware of your illness, you may continue practicing unsafe sex or other risky behaviors. Your sex or needle-sharing partner(s) may also be less likely to take precautions, since you don't appear to be ill.
3. *HIV positive, showing symptoms:* If you've been told that you have HIV and have begun showing signs or symptoms, such as swollen glands, weight loss, diarrhea, skin rashes, or others, you are at this stage. Your physical condition may gradually worsen and you may find it necessary to alter your daily activities.

4. **Acquired immune deficiency syndrome (AIDS):** This is the full-blown phase of the HIV infection. When you have AIDS, you are most prone to opportunistic infections and certain cancers. Some of the symptoms you may experience are recurrent lung infections, anemia (decreased red blood cells), more severe skin conditions such as Kaposi's sarcoma, kidney dysfunction, dementia and drastic weight loss. Nerve damage can also result in blindness, loss of hearing and difficulty walking.

Jason faces the truth

Jason decided to go to a health clinic to have his blood tested for HIV. A nurse took his blood and gave him some pamphlets to read. A doctor came in and advised Jason that it would be a good idea for him to abstain from sex while he was waiting for his test results. That was okay with Jason—he didn't really feel all that well anyway.

After a week, Jason got his test results. He had tested positive for HIV. Although the appearance of the sores on his body had hinted at a serious illness, Jason never thought he had AIDS. After all, he wasn't gay and he didn't do drugs.

Jason went back to the clinic to see if a mistake could have been made. The doctor there said that they could test him again, because false-positive test results have occurred before; however, the sores on Jason's legs looked suspiciously like Kaposi's sarcoma, a skin condition often seen among AIDS patients. Jason took another test. While waiting for his second set of test results, he suffered silently, afraid to say anything to friends, ex-girlfriends or his family. The second test results, too, came back positive for HIV.

Jason immediately met with the clinic doctor, who advised him to tell all his former or present sex partners of his blood test results. Jason says it was the hardest thing he's ever had to do in his life. Some of his previous partners took it well, while others cried, yelled at him or blamed him for putting them at risk. It was no use to rationalize with them that they had put themselves at risk as well. Jason was overcome with guilt and sincerely hoped that none of his former sex partners tested positive.

AIDS and blacks

AIDS is now one of the top ten killers in the United States. The Centers for Disease Control and Prevention (CDC), located in Atlanta, Georgia, have been keeping national statistics on AIDS patients since June 1981. The CDC estimated in 1993 that one million Americans and 12 to 15 million people worldwide were infected with HIV. Some health organizations estimate that by the year 2000, 40 million to 100 million people worldwide may be infected with HIV.

According to statistics released by the National Coalition of Black Lesbians and Gays (NCBLG), 31 percent of all Americans who have AIDS are black. What is equally if not more tragic are indications that the black family is being steadily ravaged by this disease. One out of every two women and six out of every ten children who have AIDS in the United States are black.

The CDC also reports that as of January 1, 1993, 253,448 cases of AIDS were documented in the United States. Of that number, 59,135 AIDS patients were black men over 13 years old. White males with AIDS totaled 124,827; Hispanics, 35,427; Asian/Pacific Islanders, 1,448, and Native Americans, 374.[2]

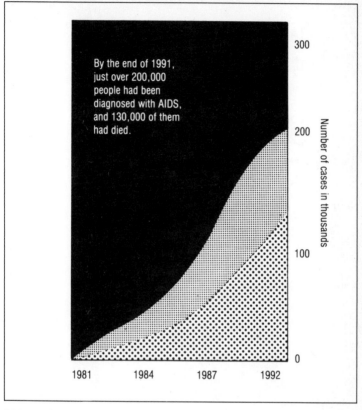

By the end of 1991, just over 200,000 people had been diagnosed with AIDS, and 130,000 of them had died.

FIGURE 9B

The growth of AIDS over a decade.
Reprinted with permission from the American Red Cross booklet "HIV and AIDS," 1992.

In the early 1980s, AIDS was viewed as a disease of gay white men. The first AIDS initiative for black people was sponsored by the CDC in October 1987. The following year, statistics indicated 31 percent of all those reported with AIDS were black. By that time, thousands of young black men and women had died and thousands more were

FACT: People with HIV live in every one of the 50 states. Everyone needs to know about HIV and AIDS. Everyone needs to learn how to prevent HIV infection.

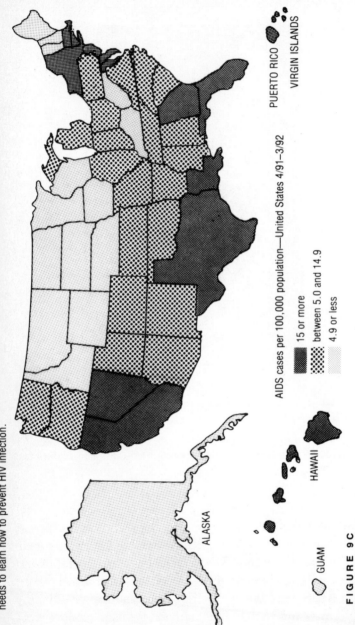

AIDS cases per 100,000 population—United States 4/91–3/92

15 or more

between 5.0 and 14.9

4.9 or less

PUERTO RICO

VIRGIN ISLANDS

ALASKA

GUAM

HAWAII

FIGURE 9C

AIDS in every state.
Reprinted with permission from the American Red Cross booklet "HIV and AIDS," 1992.

infected. "We had an epidemic on our hands," Sandra McDonald explained. McDonald is the president and founder of Outreach, Inc., a support service for people with AIDS in Atlanta, Georgia.

McDonald lowered her voice. "In the New Jersey and New York areas, hundreds of young black men were dying and everyone assumed it was from drug overdoses. In 1989, 100 bodies were exhumed. Guess what? Many of them had AIDS. By then, our black communities had already been infected and affected for a long time."

Outreach, Inc., opened its doors in 1986. McDonald ministered to the gay white community for six months before she helped her first black gay man in July 1986. "I couldn't find one," she said. "Because of the stigma attached to being gay in the black community, many homosexuals preferred being classified as IV drug users rather than gay."

McDonald said, "There has always been homosexuality in the African-American community, but we never talked about it. Why? We were aware of it, but we didn't embrace it. If we don't embrace something, we can't empower it. So instead, we have chosen to ignore homosexuality."

Sedrick Gardner, director of programs for Outreach, Inc., has worked full-time with McDonald for three years. "We are here to help everyone," said Gardner. "AIDS can be absolutely devastating. But, with society the way it is, it may very well be most difficult for a black and gay patient to deal with AIDS.

"As a black man, the gay must deal with racism every day. If he is *out of the closet,* in many cases he must learn to live without the support of his family, so he must rely on the support of close friends, if he has them. If he is open about his homosexuality in his personal life, but not with his coworkers, he may constantly live with the fear that someone at work will find out. If he has chosen to live the *straight life,* then he may be hounded continually by the universal aunt who can't understand why he isn't married yet.

"When this man comes home from work, he must remove masks and peel back layers of his persona to find himself. He has to suffer all of this because society has chosen to judge him strictly by a sex act, and not as a whole person. So many black men are dying from high blood pressure, heart disease, stress, homicide, and now it's AIDS. We've lost one generation to war, drugs and crime. We're about to lose another to AIDS."

Historically, ministers in black churches would not discuss any type of sexuality. The subject was taboo. But national efforts by Rev. Joseph E. Lowery, president of the Southern Christian Leadership Conference, and his declaration that AIDS is a "civil rights issue" for blacks, have encourged other ministers to become more involved. Many large black churches have had AIDS ministries since the late 1980s. The work of these ministries includes providing meals daily for people with AIDS, implementing buddy programs to provide emotional support and establishing housing programs.

John Templeton, director of AIDS education at Grady Memorial Hospital in Atlanta, shared a frightening statistic. "When I came here five years ago, the AIDS clinic at the hospital was located in a small, dark corner, and patients had to wait two to three weeks for an appointment. Now we are in a big, new building, on two floors, and patients must wait three months for an appointment." Approximately 3,500 patients with HIV/AIDS are followed at Grady; half are black men. In 1992, 550 of the AIDS patients being followed at the hospital died.

McDonald and others insist that things are getting better in the black community for gays and intravenous drug users. Those who cross the threshold of Outreach, Inc., receive warmth, love and acceptance. They also receive education, pamphlets and counseling. "There is no cure," said McDonald. "The only weapon we have to fight AIDS with is education."

Jason investigates the cause of his HIV infection

Jason found it very difficult to tell his past sexual partners he had been diagnosed with HIV. During one such conversation, an old girlfriend confided that she, too, had been diagnosed with HIV several years before. Perhaps he had gotten the AIDS virus from unprotected sex with her. He would probably never know. What he did know was that when he was sleeping with her, he did not use condoms regularly. Sure, if either of them had a condom at the time, he would put it on. But sometimes he forgot to bring one. Neither of them ever stopped their passion to go out and buy a condom. Now Jason wished that he had.

Am I at risk?

Anyone can get AIDS. Period. You don't have to be a male homosexual to contract HIV. In fact, the number of documented cases of AIDS in homosexuals is decreasing annually, while the number of heterosexuals testing positive for HIV is rising steadily. By simply letting your guard down one time, you can get this fatal disease.

"AIDS is a serious epidemic," said Templeton. "Anyone who has shared needles or who has been sexually active during the last ten years needs an HIV test. There are ways for those who are HIV positive to improve the quality of their lives. But before they can seek help, they need to know if they are infected."

CDC documentation indicates that HIV, the virus that causes AIDS, has been in the United States since at least 1978. Although homosexual men were historically the first group associated with AIDS, the heterosexual community is quickly catching up. The CDC has compiled a list of questions to help you determine if you're at risk of becoming infected with HIV.[3] If any of the following known risk factors apply to you, consider being tested.

- If you are a male, have you had sex with other males?
- Have you shared needles or syringes to inject drugs?
- Have you had sex with someone who may have been infected with HIV?
- Have you had a sexually transmitted disease?
- Did you receive blood transfusions or blood products between 1978 and 1985?
- Have you had sex with someone who could answer yes to any of the above questions?
- Have you had unprotected sex with someone whose HIV status you do not know?

How can I become infected by HIV?

In order for HIV to be passed from another person to you, the virus must be carried from inside the infected person's body to the inside of your body, and then to your bloodstream. This can happen through an open wound or one of the many openings in your body. Often, the virus will first enter through one of your mucous membranes, and then pass to your nearby blood vessels.

HIV can be transmitted by a variety of fluids to your

body, such as blood, semen, secretions from the vagina and cervix, and breast milk. In some HIV-infected individuals, traces of the virus have been found in tears, urine, saliva and feces, but in insufficient quantities to transmit the infection to another person. Feces and urine pose a risk only if blood is present. HIV is most concentrated in semen, blood, and vaginal and cervical secretions.

Transmission of blood

Have you noticed that your dentist now wears rubber gloves, goggles or glasses and a surgical mask while he or she works on your teeth? Have you noticed that a professional or college basketball game stops if a player gets injured and starts bleeding? The player then has to change the part of the uniform that has blood on it, the blood must be wiped up from the floor, and the floor is cleaned with a disinfectant. This procedure may seem overly cautious, but people are wising up to the dangers of getting HIV through blood.

It's dangerous to come in contact with someone else's blood. You have no idea whether or not that person is infected with HIV or other germs that may be transmitted through blood. We often have openings on our skin in the form of tiny cuts and splits, most commonly around our fingernails. Blood can, although very rarely, enter these openings, carrying HIV with it. The chances are remote, but it is possible to become infected in this way.

Some infected drug users don't care whether or not the needles they use are clean, so now many of them are infected with HIV, or have AIDS. If one drug user out of five has HIV and shares the needle with his or her other four friends, he or she is thoughtlessly spreading the virus at a rapid pace.

At one time, having a blood transfusion or organ transplant was risky. Since HIV wasn't discovered until 1983, neither blood donors nor organ donors were tested for the disease. As a result, some people who required blood transfusions in the late 1970s and early 1980s acquired the disease through the blood of donors with AIDS. Arthur Ashe, for example, acquired the HIV virus from a blood transfusion during heart surgery. Likewise, some people who had been given a second chance to live through an organ donation were unfortunately infected with HIV as a result.

Today, the chance of getting HIV through a blood transfusion is remote. Since 1985, screening of blood and organs for HIV has become very strict. Donating blood is safe. New needles are used for each donor, and all blood is tested for the HIV virus before being used with a patient. Even so, you should not donate blood if you are at high risk of having HIV. If you want to know if you have HIV, get tested at a clinic or by a doctor. Do not donate blood in order to be tested for the virus.

Exposure to semen

Semen ejaculates from your penis during orgasm. A person with an HIV infection may have a high concentration of HIV in his semen. HIV can also be found in the pre-ejaculatory fluid that comes from the tip of the penis. During unprotected vaginal intercourse, HIV from the semen can go across the mucous membrane of the vagina or cervix and can travel through the membrane to tiny blood vessels found nearby. Any abrasions or breaks in the membrane make transmission of the virus even more likely. During vaginal intercourse, the woman (the receptor) is the one most at risk.

Anal intercourse seems to be the most risky form of sex when it comes to getting HIV. As in the vagina, there is a mucous membrane in the rectum that can serve as a passageway, enabling the highly concentrated HIV found in semen to travel to the receptor's bloodstream. The rectum is designed less well than the vagina to block passage of the virus. Also, the rectum tends to have more small tears than the vaginal membrane. During anal intercourse the receptor, whether male or female, is the one most at risk.

HIV may also be transmitted through oral sex, since the mouth is lined with mucous membranes. If you have breaks or small cuts in the skin of your mouth, your risk of contracting the virus from an oral sex partner increases. During vaginal, anal and oral intercourse, using a condom or dental dam will help prevent you or your partner from acquiring HIV.

Contact with vaginal and cervical secretions

Secretions from the vagina and cervix can carry HIV, although concentrations of the virus are generally not as high as in semen and blood. Use of a condom is important because it can help protect the male from getting HIV from the female, as well as protect the female from getting HIV and other sexually transmitted diseases from the male.

Pregnancy

There is an approximately 25–30 percent chance that a pregnant woman with HIV can pass the virus to her unborn child through her blood, or, after the child is born, through breast feeding. Women who are HIV positive should discuss with a doctor the risk of passing their infection on to a baby.

Ways you cannot get HIV

It is as important for you to know how you cannot get HIV as to know how you can contract the virus. The National Coalition of Black Lesbians and Gays (NCBLG) offers the following list of ways you *cannot* become infected:

- You cannot get HIV from sitting on a toilet seat.
- You cannot get HIV from eating food prepared by someone who has the virus.
- You cannot get HIV from holding, hugging or touching a person who has the virus.
- You cannot get HIV from swimming in a pool with someone who has the virus.
- You cannot get HIV from working with or attending school with someone who has the virus.
- You cannot get HIV from a mosquito bite.
- Although a very small amount of HIV has been found in tears, saliva, urine and feces, there have been no documented cases of anyone getting the disease through transmission of these fluids because the concentration of HIV in these fluids is too low.

What complications can I develop if I have AIDS?

AIDS can affect virtually every part of your body. Changes in your skin, major organs, weight and energy level are the most obvious examples of this. The complications you experience will, for the most part, be a result of your immune system getting weaker, opening the door to other diseases.

Your immune system will be affected

Your body's immune system is made up of a variety of organs and cells, which work to rid your body of foreign substances, such as bacteria and viruses. Some of the white blood cells in your immune system, known as *CD4, T cells, T4 cells,* or *helper lymphocytes* (all different names for the same cell), normally assist your immune system in fighting disease. If you have HIV, these cells are killed for reasons not completely understood.

If you don't have HIV, your CD4 cell level is usually above 500 cells per cubic millimeters of blood. (This number indicates the amount of CD4 cells in your body.) For the AIDS patient, this number usually declines as the virus gains a foothold. As of 1993, you are considered to have AIDS by the medical community when your CD4 level dips below 200.[4] Once this happens, you may be put on preventive medicines such as Bactrim, which can help prevent infections that your immune system can no longer fight. You may also be offered one or more drugs that act directly on the HIV to reduce its impact on your body. These drugs go by the strange acronyms of *AZT, ddl, ddC* and *+ d4T.* If you are HIV positive, your CD4 count should be monitored every four to six months.

Some germs will take advantage of a low CD4 cell concentration or weakened immune system, and cause infections and disease. These include a variety of fungal, parasitic and viral infections, and certain unusual bacterial infections, such as tuberculosis (TB). In fact, TB is becoming a major problem among people who are infected with HIV.

You may develop skin disorders

Sometimes patients with AIDS, like Jason, will develop skin disorders, such as Kaposi's sarcoma, a rare cancer.

Kaposi's sarcoma can appear in all shapes, sizes and colors on your skin, though it usually appears as bruising or blotching. It can also appear anywhere inside or outside your body. Other types of skin disorders that are prevalent among AIDS patients include herpes (a viral infection, which presents itself as blisters) and psoriasis (skin lesions that appear as thickened red areas covered by white scales on your skin). Another common skin problem among HIV patients is a rash that appears on your scalp, face and neck.

You may develop a pneumocystis carinii pneumonia (PCP) infection

PCP, a lung disorder caused by a special class of bacteria, was rare before the AIDS epidemic. If you have HIV, the PCP infection can more easily cause disease because of your weakened immune system. Symptoms of PCP are shortness of breath, a cough and fever. Approximately 60 to 80 percent of all AIDS patients contract this disorder. There are a variety of medications available to treat this type of pneumonia.

You may lose weight

One of the symptoms of HIV infection is progressive weight loss. The human immunodeficiency virus causes your body to burn energy at a higher rate than normal. If you are HIV positive, you will need to increase your calorie intake and use vitamin supplements to keep up with the drastic changes your body is experiencing. (Not all HIV-positive people have this problem.)

Other HIV-related factors that have to do with weight loss are diarrhea and malnutrition. Diarrhea can be a side effect of prescription medication, a sign of serious infection or simply a symptom of HIV. Whatever the source, if you have diarrhea for more than a few days, you should notify your doctor. Diarrhea can cause dehydration, which can lead to other serious health problems. In severe cases of diarrhea, you may experience malnutrition because your food passes through your digestive system too quickly for nutrients to be properly absorbed.

Your kidneys may fail

HIV/AIDS can cause your kidneys to malfunction. Because the human immunodeficiency virus breaks down your body's immune system, every other body system can be affected. If your kidneys become infected, a variety of life-threatening disorders can occur. Read Chapter Eight for more specific information about kidney failure.

You may lose your sight

Because of nerve damage caused by HIV-related infections (specifically, an opportunistic virus called CMV), you can lose your sight to this disease. Some opportunistic infections may take advantage of your weakened system and cause a condition called retinitis, which can lead to blindness. If this disease is caught early enough, it can be treated.

Jason takes charge of his fate

Once Jason was certain he had AIDS, he went through the motions of his everyday life. He went to work, came home and kept to himself. He was feeling sorry for himself and didn't want others to watch. One day a coworker, a friend of Jason's, asked Jason if he was feeling well. The coworker could tell he had lost a lot of weight and knew that he had used several of his sick days. Jason, tired of the solitude, confided in his friend, telling him of his diagnosis. "What are you doing about it?" the coworker asked. The question caught Jason off guard. After all, everyone knows there's no cure for AIDS. "Nothing," Jason responded with a shrug.

The next day, his friend approached him with an armful of pamphlets, magazine articles and library books concerning the treatment of HIV/AIDS. After work, the two men pored over all the information, learning about the various forms of treatments. Today, Jason takes several prescription drugs to help control the complications of HIV and he's also waiting to be called to participate in a clinical trial.

You can participate in clinical trials

A clinical trial is a test of a new drug on people with HIV. When a research laboratory develops a new drug for AIDS patients, there is no way to know how the drug will work or what the side effects will be. First, the drug is tested in a test tube in the laboratory, then on animals. After that, human volunteers are needed. Since there's no cure for AIDS or HIV, many volunteers feel as though they have nothing to lose by trying an experimental drug. Some of these investigational drugs have been very helpful for people who participate in these trials. Before participating in a drug trial, you will be given lots of information about the potential risks and benefits of the drug you will be taking. You will also be carefully screened before being allowed to participate.

Remember, if you decide to participate, there's no guarantee of recovery. The drug or treatment being tested may not work at all, or may even make your condition worse. You have to decide if it's worth the risk to you. You can leave the trial and stop taking the treatment at any time. If you are interested in finding out whether you might be a candidate for a clinical trial, you can call the AIDS Treatment Data Network at (212) 268-4196. Unfortunately, many trials are very limited and can accommodate only a fraction of the number of interested persons.

AIDS support

If you are infected with HIV, support is essential. It's hard enough to cope with the disease, much less cope with it alone. There are many hotline services, outreach programs and support systems available to lend you support.

Sandra McDonald's Outreach, Inc., is an example of one. "We don't point fingers here," said McDonald. "Everyone who walks through our door is a family member." Located on the southwest side of Atlanta, Outreach, Inc., exemplifies the type of grass-roots programs being started in major cities throughout the country. These programs fill a need, which the black community has long ignored.

"People I had known all my life avoided me when I started this organization," McDonald said. "For years I rented space in downtown Atlanta because I couldn't get space in this part of town. Those damn bastards thought they would get the disease."

Sedrick Gardner facilitates several workshops at Outreach, Inc., for black men who are HIV positive. "I've seen life just turn around for some of these men," he said. "In a group, they learn to help themselves and each other. They come from all walks of life—lawyers, teachers, accountants, musicians and clerks. If you ran into the group on the street, you would never think it was an HIV support group. I've learned a lot from these men. AIDS is about life. It is not about death. Men suffering with this disease know what is important and live each day to the fullest. All of us could learn something from them."

If you would like information about services like Outreach, Inc., which are available throughout the country, call the AIDS Hotline, given at the end of this chapter. The person who answers your call will be happy to provide you with the information you need.

SECTION TWO:
SEXUALLY TRANSMITTED DISEASES

Billy has a dilemma

Billy was 18 years old and had been sexually active for the past three years. He was crazy about his new girlfriend, Kellie, and Billy knew that he was the first boy with whom she had ever been intimate. How was he going to explain to his father and his girlfriend that he had probably given her gonorrhea and she needed to be examined right away?

Other sexually transmitted diseases

If you have been diagnosed with a sexually transmitted disease (STD), HIV or otherwise, you should tell your partners. All of them. There are many sexually transmitted diseases in addition to HIV infection, of which you should be aware. Like HIV, these infections spread from one person to another during sexual contact.

According to *Healthy People 2000: National Health Promotion and Disease Prevention Objectives,* until recently only five sexually transmitted diseases were regularly monitored by the medical community. Now the number has increased dramatically in both complexity and scope, and more than 50 organisms and syndromes are recognized.[5]

While most of these diseases have been known for a long time, new diagnostic methods have helped investigators describe their extent, method of transmission and clinical consequences. Almost 12 million cases of STD occur annually in the United States. Eighty-six percent of these cases occur in people between the ages of 15 and 29. By age 21, approximately one out of every five young Americans requires treatment for a sexually transmitted disease. The total societal cost of sexually transmitted diseases exceeds $3.5 billion annually.

Anyone can contract a sexually transmitted disease— the rich, poor, young, old, black or white. If you have sexual contact with anyone with an STD, it is possible to catch it.

Gonorrhea

Gonorrhea is a localized infection involving your genitals and urinary tract. If you have contact with an infected person, you may experience gonorrhea symptoms within two to 14 days. Your symptoms may include genital discharge and burning when urinating. These symptoms are more easily recognized by men, but often go unnoticed by both men and women. Gonorrhea continues to be the most frequently reported communicable disease in the United States. The good thing about gonorrhea is that it can be treated. Since 1981, the number of men diagnosed with gonorrhea has decreased by 29 percent; the number of women, by 24 percent. However, gonorrhea has not declined among racial and ethnic minorities, or among teenagers.

A major barrier to further gonorrhea reduction is the expected increase in antibiotic-resistant strains. The proportion of all gonorrhea organisms that are antibiotic-resistant grew from .08 percent in 1985 to 7.0 percent in 1989. If gonorrhea cannot be cured by antibiotics or is antibiotic-resistant, it can cause sterility, arthritis, blindness or damage to your urinary tract. If a pregnant woman has gonorrhea, it can also cause blindness in her unborn child.[6]

Syphilis

Syphilis affects your entire body system and has the potential to do even more damage than gonorrhea. There are three stages in the development of syphilis. In the primary stage, a painless sore or chancre appears at the place where the germ first entered your body. This usually occurs on the genitals and can happen within three months after contact with an infected person. This chancre can go unnoticed, especially in women, and will disappear on its own with or without treatment, as the disease goes into the next stage.

The secondary stage of syphilis is characterized by skin rashes, hair loss, sore throat, fever and headaches, all of which will disappear on their own. In the final stage, the disease goes deeper into your body until it reappears years later after doing irreparable damage. Untreated, syphilis can cause blindness, deafness, heart disease, insanity and eventually, death. Women who have the disease when they are pregnant may give birth to children who are handicapped or stillborn. Like gonorrhea, syphilis can also be treated with antibiotics.

Herpes simplex

Herpes simplex is a virus that affects your genitourinary system. Symptoms appear from two to 20 days after you have had contact with an infected partner. You may experience one or groups of small bumps or blisters in your genital area—on, around or inside the vagina, on the penis, in or around the anus. These blisters can be very painful and uncomfortable, and you may also feel ill. The blisters usually begin to dry up and disappear within five to 20 days.

There is no cure for herpes, but there is treatment. You can infect another person anytime, even when your symptoms are not present. When the blisters disappear, the virus remains in your body, and symptoms may recur when you are rundown, have a cold, fever, are tired, sunburned, emotionally upset or suffering from stress. A medicine called acylovir can ease the symptoms, decrease the duration of the attack, and help prevent recurrences. But, again, there is no cure for herpes.

Venereal warts

Venereal warts are also caused by a virus. The symptoms usually develop 30 to 90 days after you have had contact with an infected partner. These small warts can appear anywhere in and around the penis, vagina or anus. They don't usually hurt or itch, and may go unnoticed unless you look for them or discover them by touch.

As long as you have symptoms, you are infectious. Even after the warts disappear, the virus remains in your body, and may recur when you are rundown. There is no cure for venereal warts, but they can be managed by freezing or burning them off.

Chlamydia

Of all the infectious diseases mentioned here, chlamydia is probably the least known among the general population, yet paradoxically, is the most frequent sexually transmitted germ in the U.S. *Healthy People 2000* researchers estimate that four million acute infections occur annually from this organism. Many people with the disease have no symptoms or signs of infection. Inflammation of the male urethra, the duct that transports urine from the bladder through the prostate and penis, is called urethritis. Thirty to 50 percent of these infections are caused by the chlamydia microorganism. Chlamydia can be treated. However, many doctors claim that because there are not many affordable diagnostic tests for the disease, it's difficult to diagnose chlamydia patients who are not experiencing obvious symptoms. Also, many patients who must undergo the current seven-day medication treatment do not complete their regimen. Fortunately, a one-dose treatment is being tested that may be equally effective. The advantage of a single-dose treatment is that patients are more likely to complete treatment, and thus are more likely to be cured before having sexual intercourse again.[7]

Other infections

There are some common vaginal infections that women can contract and pass on to a partner. These include bacterial infections, yeast, fungal or trichomonas infections. Some of the symptoms of these infections include discharge, itching, a foul odor, painful or frequent urination, dryness and sensitivity around and inside the vagina. In addition, men often get infections that produce discharge, painful or frequent urination and sensitivity to the penis. These infections can also be passed on to a partner.

Pubic lice and scabies

Pubic lice, commonly called crabs, are animals about the size of a pinhead that live in the hairy areas of your genitals and other hairy parts of your body. Some people experience intense itching or rashes while others, who are not allergic to the lice bite, may not experience symptoms. Crabs can be cured by applying a specially prescribed medicated soap or shampoo.

Scabies are mites that can cause itchy rashes or small raised reddish tracts anywhere on your skin's surface. These are transmitted venereally and through close body contact and are highly infectious. Your doctor can prescribe a number of different creams or lotions to cure scabies.

A special note about tuberculosis

Tuberculosis is not considered a "sexually transmitted disease" because it is airborne. Moreover, it has been in decline for decades. Not too long ago, physicians and medical professionals were congratulating each other on the supposed elimination of tuberculosis (TB) in the U.S. Now, however, the entire United States is experiencing the worst epidemic of tuberculosis since the 1960s. In New York City, a drug-resistant strain of tuberculosis killed 12 inmates and a prison guard. Some health care workers have also died from this strain, and as a result, a New York City task force has recommended instituting new TB-screening measures.

According to an article in *The Journal of The American Medical Association (JAMA)*,[8] the United Hospital Fund of New York published a report in December 1992 on the resurgence of tuberculosis in AIDS patients. In New York City, 600,000 to 1,000,000 people were infected with tuberculosis in 1993, and 40 percent of those with TB were also infected with HIV. The Centers for Disease Control and Prevention has included TB as a common infection associated with AIDS.

If you suspect that you have been exposed to TB bacteria, you should have a tuberculin skin test immediately. If the test is positive, you can get a chest X ray and laboratory test to determine the level of the disease in your system. As we mentioned earlier, tuberculosis is an airborne disease, which means it spreads when a person with tuberculosis coughs or sneezes and sends the tubercle bacilli (bacterium that causes tuberculosis) germs into the air. You become infected with TB when you inhale these germs.

Symptoms include a chronic cough, fatigue, weakness, night sweats, drastic weight loss, blood in your sputum and low-grade fever. The disease is treated with antibiotics; a course of drug therapy for at least six months will protect your lungs from any permanent damage.

Conclusion

The most important thing to remember about AIDS and other STDs is that you can avoid every disease and infection (except perhaps tuberculosis) mentioned in this chapter. The best way to avoid becoming infected with

HIV (the virus that causes AIDS), as well as other sexually transmitted diseases, is by avoiding the high-risk behaviors listed in this chapter. While condoms alone do not provide complete protection, they do reduce your chance of being infected with HIV, as well as many other infections.

Use condoms properly and every time you have sex—vaginal, anal or oral. You can also prevent an HIV infection by abstaining from sex completely or having sex with only one mutually faithful, uninfected partner, and by not sharing needles. Remember, if you take precautions, sexually transmitted infections don't have to be a part of your life.

If you suspect you have been exposed to someone infected with HIV or an STD, remember—these infections are very common and are nothing to be embarrassed about. See a medical professional immediately, because early treatment can help to prevent long-term damage. Continue following the guidelines in this chapter to ensure that you are getting the greatest care possible and preventing others from also becoming infected. Remember, you are the most important player when it comes to your own health care.

Resources

The American Red Cross
2025 E Street N.W.
Washington, DC 20009
(202) 728-6400

(Contact your local chapter for resources, programs, brochures on AIDS, training classes and services.)

Centers for Disease Control and Prevention (CDC)
1600 Clifton Road, N.E.
Atlanta, Georgia 30333
(404) 332-4555

(This organization provides information through telephone voice messages, fax machines or the mail.)

The Department of Public Health

(Contact your local or state department of public health for HIV and AIDS information.)

National AIDS Hotline
(800) 342-2437
(800) 342-AIDS
(800) 243-7889 (For persons with hearing
    impairments)

(When you call the hotline, staff members will answer your questions regarding AIDS. They will also send brochures when requested and make referrals. This also applies to the SIDA hotline, below.)

National Association of People With AIDS
1413 K Street N.W.
Washington, DC 20005
(202) 898-0414

(This group provides supportive services to AIDS patients. When you call, they will put you in touch with local chapters.)

National Institute of Allergy and Infectious
    Diseases (NIAID)
AIDS Clinical Trials Information Service

PO Box 6421
Rockville, MD 20849-6421
(800) 874-2572
(800) TRIALS-A

(This service offers clinical trial information.)

Retrovir Prescription Program for AIDS Patients
Pharmacy Management Services
3611 Queen Palm Drive
Tampa, FL 33619
(800) 237-7676, Ext. 6617

(This program provides medication at wholesale prices, for HIV patients exclusively. Medicine can be delivered overnight by Federal Express.)

The Rotary Club

(The Rotary Club in Los Altos, California, has produced an educational videotape about HIV and AIDS called "The Los Altos Story." Contact your local Rotary Club for information on obtaining the tape.)

SIDA National AIDS Hotline (Spanish)
(800) 344-7432
(800) 344-SIDA

State Agencies

(Look up AIDS under "state agencies" in your local phone book to find out about financial aid programs.)

10

Substance Abuse

Nathan errs in judgment

Nathan worked at a local newspaper as a reporter. After work, before heading home to his wife and children, he always used to stop at the local bar, where he would meet some of his friends. Nathan always looked forward to this break in the day. He thought of himself as a social drinker. "Just a few drinks with the gang and then I'd head home for a late dinner," he said. "I never thought the alcohol really affected me."

One evening, however, after his normal three double scotches, Nathan got into his car to head home. A light rain was beginning to fall. Just as he was approaching his neighborhood, he accidentally sped through a red light going south. An eastbound car sideswiped him. Nathan's car spun around, hit a parked car, and then landed on the porch of one of his neighbors' homes. When the police arrived, they administered a sobriety test. Nathan *failed. Blood tests indicated he was over the legal limit for alcohol in his system.*

Fortunately, no one was hurt and only property damage was incurred, but the incident was enough to shake up Nathan. It took a while, but he finally admitted he was an alcoholic and joined Alcoholics Anonymous. Nathan now knows that there is no such thing as an ex-alcoholic. He will always be recovering, but never cured.

What is substance abuse?

Almost all Americans are guilty of substance abuse of one kind or another. Think about how many people you know who have to have a cup of coffee in the morning to get themselves going. As consumers, we are constantly inundated with advertisements for beer, caffeine, pain-killers, cigarettes—things that will "make us feel better." We're constantly being told that we just need that "little something"—whether it's a cigarette, drug or drink—and all our problems will be solved. What these ads fail to tell you is that unless you feel good about yourself, and respect yourself enough to treat your body right, your problems will persist.

Simply put, substance abuse is the misuse or nonmedical use of drugs, alcohol or tobacco products. We are guilty of abuse whenever we use substances to alter our moods, self-perceptions or environments. The effects of substance abuse touch virtually all of us in America today, either directly or indirectly. Abuse becomes an addiction when you develop a physical or psychological dependency on your substance of choice. If you find yourself thinking, "I just have to have one more cigarette . . . cup of coffee . . . drink . . . joint . . .or upper," there's a good chance you're an addict.

No matter what you're addicted to, breaking yourself of a habit is never easy. It's important to be patient with yourself, set small attainable goals, and take it day by day, hour by hour, minute by minute. When trying to break yourself of an addiction (and most of us are addicted to *something* at some point in our lives), professional help is often necessary. There are many resources available to make your challenge easier. Remember—you are not alone.

Anyone can be a substance abuser. Everyone is at risk, whether black, white, male, female, old, middle-aged or a child in elementary school. Professionals, blue-collar workers, athletes, movie stars, the poor and the rich—all these people fit the profile. In fact, contrary to common belief, approximately 70 percent of all substance abusers are employed.

The effects of substance abuse are tearing apart our workplaces, homes, schools and families. Substance abuse begins for many different reasons. Some of us may turn to alcohol or drugs at a young age because of peer pressure. We all know how difficult it can be to say no when we're trying to feel accepted by the very people who are pushing us to do something. As adults, we may turn to a substance to ease ourselves of depression, mental anguish, or pressure from home or work. Some of us may turn to drugs like amphetamines (speed) to keep us "up," believing that we can be more productive at work. Still others of us, like Nathan, may turn to alcohol or drugs because it helps us relax and is a way to socialize.

Choosing whether or not to take drugs, consume alcohol or use tobacco is a decision we each must make at some time or another. We may rationalize that the substances we use affect only us, therefore it's no one else's business. However, everyone is at risk when, like Nathan, you get behind the wheel of a car after drinking or when a drug addict turns to crime to support his or her habit, or when a smoker puts his family at risk of lung cancer because of secondhand smoke.

Substance abuse and blacks

Just as within any community, abuse of alcohol and drugs creates great problems within the black community. Substance abuse can lead to physical and mental health problems, a lack of education, unemployment, crime and violence.

Two blacks to every one white die from cirrhosis of the liver, which is caused primarily by alcoholism.[1] Blacks between the ages of 25 and 34 have a 10 percent greater chance of dying from cirrhosis than their white counterparts.[2] Black males die three times more often than white men from esophageal cancer, which is believed to be caused by the combined abuse of alcohol and tobacco.

"Blacks are three times more likely to be in treatment for a drug abuse–related problem than whites," reads the *Report of the Secretary's Task Force on Black & Minority Health*.[3] This report used data obtained from the 1982 National Drug and Alcoholism Treatment Utilization Survey (NDATUS). The statistics speak for themselves. Alcohol, drug abuse and tobacco use are practically tearing the black community apart.

Nationwide, however, substance abuse seems to be decreasing somewhat. This may be because the social climate has changed greatly from the late sixties and early seventies. Statistics released from the *Third Triennial Report to Congress from the Secretary, Department of Health and Human Services, on Drug Abuse and Drug Abuse Research* indicate that drug use in the United

States, while still high, has decreased sharply from the epidemic levels seen in the 1970s. For example:

- Marijuana has been used, at one time or another, by a third of all Americans. However, the percentage who reported currently using it in the month preceding the 1988 National Household Survey decreased to 5.9 percent compared to 9 percent reporting use in 1985.
- In 1988, 12-to-17-year-olds were drinking and smoking less than those of the same age in 1985. Approximately 25 percent of the group—down from 31 percent—had consumed alcohol in the month preceding the 1988 survey. The number of smokers in this age group also decreased: 11.8 percent were current smokers, while in 1985, 15.3 percent claimed to be.
- More than one-third (35.2 percent) of young adults still smoke. However, the percentage of adults older than age 26 who smoke (29.8 percent) is only three-quarters as large as it was in 1974.[4]

Alcohol and blacks

When it comes to alcohol problems, blacks are disproportionately affected. Sadly enough, the number of us who have medical problems as a result of heavy drinking has increased in recent years. Years ago, rates of acute and chronic alcohol-related diseases among blacks were lower than or similar to those for whites. Recently, however, these rates have increased. Currently, we are at high risk for developing acute and chronic alcohol-related diseases including alcoholic fatty liver, hepatitis, liver cirrhosis and esophageal cancer (as mentioned above).[5]

Another major difference in black versus white drinking patterns appears to be the ages at which we begin and stop drinking heavily. Among white males, heavy and problematic drinking is most evident among young men. Black men, on the other hand, are more likely to demonstrate problematic drinking habits in middle age, usually after age 30. This pattern of late onset, if it leads to prolonged, heavy consumption, may put us at greater risk for chronic diseases related to alcohol consumption.

What is alcoholism?

A simple definition of alcoholism is addiction to ethyl alcohol. Approximately 10 percent of all drinkers become alcoholics. The other 90 percent are not alcoholic. If you're trying to determine if you are addicted to alcohol, you may find the following medically defined distinctions helpful.

Occasional drinker: If you are an occasional drinker, you drink alcohol on rare occasions. Even then, you drink only sparingly. Alcohol is not a major part of your daily life and, as a result, has never been a problem for you.

Frequent drinker: If you are a frequent drinker, you may have a couple drinks at parties or among friends because it makes you feel good. You rarely, however, drink enough to get drunk. People in this group are sometimes referred to as "social drinkers."

Regular drinker: As a regular drinker, you consider drinking an important part of your life. However, you could give up drinking if necessary.

Heavy drinker: If you're a heavy drinker, alcohol is a problem in your life. This means you are alcohol-dependent and cannot easily handle social situations without having a drink. You could give up alcohol only with great difficulty, which means you are prone to becoming an alcoholic. If you fall in this group, it would be worth your while to seek help or try to cut down on your alcohol intake.

Alcoholic: An alcoholic is a heavy drinker who has lost control over his or her alcohol consumption. If you're an alcoholic, you cannot function at work, home or in a social setting without a drink. You also can't stop at one drink. Your alcohol abuse may change your personality drastically, and even cause you to have blackouts on occasion. You may even have lost interest in eating or suffer from severe weight loss. It's important to realize that the effects of alcoholism differ among alcoholics, depending on body chemistry or eating habits.

If you are an alcoholic, a constant threat in your life may be alcohol withdrawal. In other words, if you go too long without having a drink, or if you're trying to become sober or break the addiction, you may experience the "shakes," or hallucinations. During the hallucinations, called delirium tremens, or DTs, you may imagine that you see insects, spiders or other bugs, which seem to be missing their legs. You may also imagine that there are animals in the room with you, probably because you misinterpret shadows and sounds. People may tell you that you're talking compulsively or indistinctly, and your arms and legs may shake, because of muscle twitches and spasms.

These delirium tremens may be caused by an altered brain function brought about by alcohol abuse, especially among those who have been excessive and steady drinkers for many years, or who are recovering from a recent drinking binge. Current research suggests that DTs may result from a biochemical disorder in your brain.

Sometimes DT symptoms may be accompanied by fever which can get high enough to cause your circulatory system to collapse. About 15 percent of those who experience DTs die because of shock or circulatory collapse. DTs are considered to be a medical emergency. If you experience DTs or are ever with someone who does, seek medical assistance immediately. Large amounts of water are often given intravenously, so that the sodium, potassium and magnesium added to it can replace those minerals lost in the perspiration that accompanies high fever. Muscle tremors may be treated with tranquilizing drugs. DTs usually end within approximately two days.

Alcoholism not only affects us physically, but also has severe social consequences. Recent statistics show that driving under the influence of alcohol accounts for half of all fatal motor vehicle accidents in the United States. An increasing number of reported industrial accidents, crimes of violence against adults and children, housebreakings, and robberies involve alcohol use. In addition, the number of juvenile alcoholics seems to be increasing. These youngsters, as well as adults, also mix alcohol with other drugs—especially cocaine.

Treating the alcoholic

According to Peter Bell, the director of the Institute on Black Chemical Abuse in Minneapolis, black individuals and families tend to seek help for alcohol problems later in the progression of the illness than their white counterparts. As a consequence, black families may be significantly more dysfunctional and resistant to messages of recovery than white families.

Alcoholics Anonymous (AA) is one group that tries to help alcoholics help themselves. The philosophy of this group is "once an alcoholic, always an alcoholic," but you can control the disease through determination, the support of other recovering alcoholics and, of course, by not drinking. AA has developed Twelve Steps (see below) and a buddy system to help you to sobriety. There are also several groups that have been developed for relatives or friends of alcoholics. These include Al-Anon and Alateen, a program for teenagers whose parents are alcoholics.

Twelve Steps

The following Twelve Steps are established by Alcoholics Anonymous to help alcoholics break their addiction. The idea of AA is that the addict will make these steps a way of life. No matter what you are addicted to, you may find them to be helpful.

1. We admitted we were powerless over alcohol—that our lives had become unmanageable.
2. Came to believe that a Power greater than ourselves could restore us to sanity.
3. Made a decision to turn our will and our lives over to the care of God *as we understood God to be*.
4. Made a searching and fearless moral inventory of ourselves.
5. Admitted to God, to ourselves and to another human being the exact nature of our wrongs.
6. Were entirely ready to have God remove all these defects of character.
7. Humbly asked God to remove our shortcomings.

8. Made a list of all persons we had harmed, and became willing to make amends to them all.
9. Made direct amends to such people wherever possible, except when to do so would injure them or others.
10. Continued to take personal inventory and when we were wrong promptly admitted it.
11. Sought, through prayer and meditation, to improve our conscious contact with God *as we understood God to be,* praying only for knowledge of God's will for us and the power to carry that out.
12. Having had a spiritual awakening as the result of these Steps, we tried to carry this message to others, and to practice these principles in all our affairs.[6]

Tobacco abuse

Another common substance that is abused in American society, especially among blacks, is tobacco. For more information about nicotine addiction, see Chapter Two.

Our fascination with tobacco dates way back. During his explorations, Columbus first discovered Caribbean Indians smoking leaves of the "tabaca" plant and brought the plant back to Europe. In less than 50 years, people in every major city in Europe were smoking. As early as the 1600s, governments attempted to ban the habit, and in some countries the punishment for smoking was death. Yet even with that ultimate discouragement, the number of smokers increased.

Today, 60 million Americans smoke cigarettes and more than 6 million U.S. men smoke cigars. *The Report of the Secretary's Task Force on Black Minority Health* states that "cigarette smoking is the chief preventable cause of death in the United States. Cigarette smoking is a causal factor for coronary heart disease and arterio-sclerotic peripheral vascular disease; cancer of the lung, larynx, oral cavity and esophagus; and chronic bronchitis and emphysema. It is also associated with cancer of the urinary tract, bladder, pancreas, and kidney and with ulcer disease and low birthweight."

In April 1993, the Centers for Disease Control and Prevention reported that a steady 25-year decline in smoking had leveled off. The CDC reported that 46.3 million adults (25.7 percent) smoked in 1991, compared to 25.5 percent who smoked in 1990. Their report also stated that more blacks (29.2 percent, versus 26.2 percent in 1990) smoke than any other groups.

The age at which someone first takes up smoking is crucial, according to the September 1990 issue of *the Journal of the American Medical Association (JAMA)*. Once you become an established smoker, quitting is more difficult, because nicotine is a highly addictive drug.

According to the *JAMA* article, which looked at 14,764 people ranging from ages 18 to 35 (of that group, 811 were black men), smoking begins in all racial groups as early as age nine. The incidence of starting to smoke then increases rapidly after age 11, peaking between ages 17 and 19 among all race and ethnic groups. In addition, smoking rates were generally higher for black and Hispanic men and women.[7]

Curtis listens to reason

Curtis is 70 years old and in excellent health. He's up every day at 7 A.M. for a three-mile walk. His neighbors recognize him by his white, blue and purple jumpsuit.

Fifteen years ago, Curtis could barely walk up the six steps to his bedroom in his split-level home. He smoked two packs of cigarettes a day. During a routine physical, his doctor took X rays of his lungs. The film showed lung damage, the result of 35 years of smoking. Dr. Williams told Curtis that if he didn't stop smoking, he would shorten his life considerably. It was not the first time she had told him this, but it was the first time he listened.

Previously, in Chapter Two, we mentioned the hazardous effects of smoking on the body. Tobacco use is responsible for more than one of six deaths in the United States and accounts for about 390,000 deaths yearly including 21 percent of all coronary heart disease deaths, 87 percent of lung cancer deaths, and 30 percent of all cancer deaths. In 1987, 34 percent of blacks smoked—41 percent of all black men, and 29 percent of all black women.

Smokeless tobacco

Smokeless tobacco use increased 40 percent between 1970 and 1986 and is predominately seen in young men, according to *Healthy People 2000*. Although statistics show that black men use smokeless tobacco less than whites, it's important to be aware of the risks involved with smokeless tobacco.

Oral cancer appears to occur several times more frequently among smokeless tobacco users than among nonusers, and may be 50 times as frequent among long-term snuff users. All smokeless tobacco products contain substantial amounts of nicotine, which may lead to nicotine dependence and eventual cigarette use.[8]

Treatment

If you don't smoke, don't start. If you smoke, stop! There are several methods of stopping smoking, such as nicotine patches (available only with a medical prescription), self-help classes and hypnosis, among others. Ask your doctor for specific information on how you can stop smoking. Your success relies entirely on your willingness to quit. Attitude is everything. (Refer to Chapter Two for more information about how to break your nicotine addiction.)

Other kinds of substance abuse

While alcohol and nicotine abuse may be most obvious in today's society because they are legal substances, there are many other substances whose abuse have far-reaching consequences for the black community.

Eugene's story

Eugene was a 28-year-old man who worked 12 to 16 hours a day. He had just finished law school and had been hired by a high-powered law firm that expected him to produce approximately 200 billable hours a month. Eugene expected to have to work a lot at first, so he didn't complain.

At the end of his first year at the huge law firm, Eugene and his wife, Delia purchased a four-bedroom home in an upscale suburban community outside Chicago. He had also bought Delia a new Saab. "I earned a great deal of money working all those hours," said Eugene, "but Delia and I were also spending money at a rapid rate. That made me want to work more hours, spending more nights and weekends at work."

The long hours soon began to take a toll on Eugene. He was tired all of the time and even found himself nodding off at social functions. "I was working on a Fortune

500 account when I started taking uppers to stay awake. One of the associates at my office gave me some during a particularly hairy week. I had been given a chance to prove myself by defending one of our big clients in court. I spent nearly the whole week at work, working all night and dozing off at embarrassing times during the day. I took the pills—I didn't want to lose the account or the case." Eugene didn't lose either one, but nearly lost Delia after he continued to take amphetamines every day. "It had gotten to a point where I couldn't function without the pills," Eugene said.

Drugs

When the term *drug abuse* is mentioned, the assumption is usually that the drug being abused is illegal. Not true. The abuse of prescription drugs is as frequent as the abuse of illegal drugs.

Drug abuse is the misuse or nonmedical use of drugs for the purpose of altering your mood or perception. While certain drugs are prescribed by doctors to make you feel better, many illegal drugs attack your central nervous system and cause mental instability and emotional dependency. With some drugs, physical dependency even occurs. These drugs alter your normal behavior.

Following are some of the more common types of illegal drugs that are abused.

Marijuana

Indian hemp has been known to us for at least 3,000 years. Hemp was first used for commercial purposes, such as the production of rope and textiles. It is mentioned in ancient Sanskrit literature dating from 2000 to 1400 B.C. Later, it was utilized for medicinal and anesthetic purposes by Chinese, Hindu and Arab physicians. Not until the tenth century of the Christian era was hemp used extensively, in India and Arab countries, for its intoxicant and euphoric properties.

Among the numerous forms of the drug are Indian hemp, hashish and marijuana. You may have heard marijuana cigarettes referred to as reefers, joints, weed, grass or sticks.

Whatever it's called, marijuana is a depressant that affects your central nervous system. After using marijuana, you would probably feel sedated, depressed, drowsy or sleepy. Marijuana can be taken by mouth, baked in a cake or brownies, or smoked, which is the preferred method in the United States. Marijuana cigarettes are most often hand-rolled in white or brown cigarette papers. A heavy user may smoke as many as six cigarettes a day.

When first using marijuana, you likely noticed an increase in your hunger or desire for sweets. As a regular user, you may experience the "munchies" throughout the day. Other side effects include clumsiness and poor coordination, flushing of your face and dilation of your pupils. After smoking a joint, your pulse rate and blood pressure will elevate and you may need to urinate more often.

It's very difficult to recognize a marijuana user by sight, but the drug's smoke has an easily identifiable, distinctive odor. If you smell this odor, or if someone you know seems "spacey," disconnected, or breaks into fits of inappropriate laughter, it's possible he or she is a marijuana user.

If you are a habitual marijuana user, you probably have little desire to be cured. You may believe that smoking marijuana is neither harmful nor habit-forming. But being addicted to marijuana, like any drug, is very dangerous. It may pose long-term risks to your body and it can negatively impact your relationships with those you care about. You may also find yourself to be more irritable, garrulous and complaining than you were before you began using the drug. In some cases, using marijuana may lead you to use stronger, more addictive drugs.

Phencyclidine: PCP

Angel dust, green tea, peace pill, hog, busy bee, cyclone, mist, goon, rocket fuel, crystal, super joint, zombie dust and elephant tranquilizer are just some of the street names for phencyclidine (PCP).

PCP was developed by pharmacologists for use as an anesthetic in surgery. Permission for testing the drug on human subjects was granted in 1963 by the Food and Drug Administration (FDA). Though PCP functioned well in the operating room, the aftermath of the drug was terrible. Patients regained consciousness disoriented, delirious, hallucinating and depressed. Because of these very serious effects, the FDA withdrew its approval for use with humans. It was approved, however, as an animal anesthetic.

PCP has been on the streets since 1967, when laboratories were set up to produce the drug illegally. PCP is cheap to make, and profits are high. The drug can be taken in three forms: pill, powder or liquid. One drug-abuse expert has called PCP "a drug of terror." In small doses, it gives you a free-floating feeling or numbness, the illusion that your mind has separated from your body. In large doses, it produces symptoms of schizophrenia, which can lead to suicide and violence. The drug is stored in the fat tissues of your brain, and the rate of its breakdown in your liver is very slow.

In addition to hallucinations and flashbacks, if you use PCP, you can experience drowsiness, an inability to verbalize your thoughts and difficulty in thinking. Profuse sweating, involuntary eye movements, loss of feeling of pain, double vision, lack of muscular coordination, dizziness, nausea and vomiting are all common signs of PCP use.

Lysergic acid diethylamide: LSD

LSD made its appearance in 1943. It is colorless, odorless and tasteless. A drop of LSD (too small to be seen without a magnifying glass) is all it takes to cause you to hallucinate. Also known by the nicknames acid, paper, cubes, trips, Pearly Gates and Heavenly Blue, LSD is usually dropped onto a sugar cube or a small square of paper, or is added to orange juice. LSD can also be mixed with inert materials and formed into small tablets or caplets. Shortly after you ingest LSD, you'll begin to experience physical changes. Your pupils may dilate, heart may palpitate, blood pressure may elevate and the smooth muscles of your internal organs will contract.

At first, these symptoms may seem mild. After 30 minutes, however, you will probably begin to have hallucinations. A hallucinogenic "trip" can last up to 10 hours. The horror of LSD is that if you are a user, you are not in control of yourself. You lose your good judgment, and your environment begins to seem unreal. Some users, feeling indestructible, do foolish things while on a trip. Your mood may fluctuate when under the influence of LSD, so that you feel happy at one moment and then, a minute later, fall into a deep depression.

Barbiturates

In recent years, more and more drug users have become addicted to barbiturates because of their relatively easy availability, as compared to opiates and marijuana. Opiate addicts frequently use barbiturates to tide them over when opiates are either unobtainable or in short supply. Like chronic alcoholics, barbiturate addicts may use the drug for a single night's binge, for prolonged sprees, or every day for months or years. In many cases, people use barbiturates along with alcohol or amphetamines.

Barbiturate addicts seem to prefer the more potent, rapidly active drugs, such as Nembutal and Seconal. General terms for barbiturates are goof balls and barbs. You may have also heard them referred to as yellow jackets or pink ladies—special terms that correspond to the color of the capsules. Barbiturate users generally take 1.0 to 1.5 grams daily, usually orally, though some addicts prefer the intravenous route. Barbiturates can be extremely irritating and may cause large abscesses if injected into your subcutaneous tissues.

Tyrone sells drugs

Tyrone began selling drugs when he was in his teens to support himself, his mother and his two sisters. He was a very likable young man and his teachers did everything to convince him to stay in school, but he dropped out when his father deserted his family. He found a job in the neighborhood grocery store as a butcher, but "It didn't pay enough," he said. "I made more money selling drugs for a few hours than cutting meat for a week.

"My mother didn't like it, but there was nothing she

could do about it," Tyrone said. His mother worked as a cleaning woman in a downtown office building. Tyrone told his mother that he would stop selling drugs as soon as the family was out of debt and they could get a nice place to live.

Tyrone was now a "businessman." He wore tailored suits and Italian shoes. His hands were manicured, and he drove a midnight blue convertible. He moved his mother into a new home, and he married a beautiful young woman.

Soon, Tyrone was managing a fairly large shopping center, and he and his wife were expecting their first child. He had not given up his drug connections. In fact, the scenario got worse because, in addition to selling, Tyrone had started using cocaine. It was difficult to be around it and not try it, Tyrone says now. After he tried it, he got hooked.

"It took the birth of my daughter to make me realize what I was doing to my body and to my family," Tyrone said. "My wife wouldn't let me near the baby. My nose was running, my speech was slurred, my eyes were red and I couldn't perform in the bedroom."

Tyrone became determined to get away from his drug connections and make a new life for himself and his family. He moved his family to another state where he spent three months in a treatment program. He is now a manager in a family-owned business and counsels young adults against the use of drugs.

Heroin

Heroin is a narcotic that comes from opium. An opiate (morphine or codeine, for example) is a drug that causes sleep or stupor, and at the same time relieves pain. Because opiate drugs make people insensitive to pain, they are known by the medical community as analgesic drugs and by others as pain killers. Some of the street names for heroin are "H," skag, junk, dirt, boy, horse, smack, Mexican mud and brown sugar.

The only natural source of morphine and codeine is opium. Opium comes from the poppy plant, which thrives in the hot, dry climates of Turkey, China, India, Iran and Mexico. Heroin is a semi-synthetic drug made from the morphine obtained from the stem of the poppy.

At one time, heroin addicts were thought to be found only in poor economic areas in large inner cities. But heroin has moved from ghetto alleys to upper-middle-class living rooms and the kitchens of small-town America. An investor can buy a huge amount of heroin for $1,000 in France, and then sell it wholesale in the U.S. for more than $1 million.

Heroin is usually injected into your veins, which is called "mainlining." "Skin-popping" is when you inject the liquid form of the drug under your skin. Heroin may also be taken into your body through your nose, which is known as "snorting." The user's goal is to allow the heroin to travel through his or her bloodstream, so that it reaches all cells in the body. Heroin use affects your brain cells and decreases your heartbeat and respiration rate. Have you ever wondered why heroin addicts often wear dark sunglasses, even at night? The pupils of their eyes dilate and contract because of the rise and fall of heroin in the blood. They wear glasses to hide this inappropriate dilation of their pupils.

Heroin is a highly addictive narcotic. If you are addicted to heroin, you are probably mentally and physically incapable of thinking or doing anything without the drug. It takes larger and larger doses to get the same effect, and you can become painfully ill with muscle cramps and vomiting when you do not have access to the drug.

You can tell if someone is addicted to heroin if they frequently nod off or are drowsy. This will be especially evident right after they've had a "fix." Another dead giveaway is needle tracks along arms, hands and legs. Addicts may also frequently experience ulcerated, festering sores, as a result of using dirty needles or contaminants in the heroin.

Malnutrition is a serious consequence of heroin addiction. If you are addicted, food will not appeal to you. Your only interest will be the drug. You will probably lose a great deal of weight and become very susceptible to disease. Because heroin addicts use and share dirty needles, it is also not uncommon for them to suffer from blood poisoning, hepatitis, malaria and AIDS. (See Chapter Nine for more information about AIDS.)

Cocaine

Cocaine-related deaths among blacks have tripled from 51 to 177 per 100,000 over the past three years. For whites, the number has doubled from 149 to 312.[9] Cocaine addiction is very hard to break. Just as with heroin, cocaine will cause you to "lose your conscience." If you are addicted to cocaine, you are likely to do anything to get more of the drug. Mothers who are addicted often forget to take care of their children. Addicts will give up their homes, jobs and families—getting more of the drug is their only concern.

Street names for cocaine are coke, snow, snowbirds, "C," happy dust, gold dust, flake, Cecil, stardust, Bernice, white girl, girl and speedball (which is heroin and cocaine used together). Cocaine is an odorless, sometimes crystalline or fluffy white powder. Unlike heroin or morphine, it is a stimulant. This means instead of making you sleepy, it will keep you awake.

Cocaine is usually taken into your bloodstream by one of four methods: snorting, mainlining, smoking or "skin pops." When you "snort," or take cocaine through your nose, its effect lasts a long time. When you inject it into your bloodstream through mainlining, the effect of the drug lasts only for approximately 10 minutes. It is possible for IV drug abusers to "use up" all the veins in their body through overuse. When this happens, some abusers will become so desperate that they'll do "skin pops," which means they inject the drug under the skin into capillaries just beneath the skin's surface.

Cocaine base can also be smoked, which is called freebasing. To process cocaine hydrochloride for freebasing, the drug is treated with a solution of baking soda and ether. When these are mixed together, a layer of liquid containing cocaine forms on top. This layer is removed into a separate dish, and the extra liquid is allowed to evaporate. The powder produced by this process is known as "freebase." It is put into a water pipe and heated with a propane torch to turn the cocaine into vapor. It was once publicized that comedian Richard Pryor was badly burned from an explosion of ether as he was preparing to freebase.

To avoid the inconvenience and danger of preparing cocaine for freebasing, chemists who deal in illegal drugs have developed a simpler method of changing cocaine hydrochloride into a smokable form. The result is a new drug called *crack*. (See next section.)

Regardless of how you take it, cocaine works on your central nervous system raising your pulse and respiration rates, increasing your body temperature and elevating your blood pressure. Cocaine constricts your blood vessels and dilates your pupils. The drug induces a kind of hyperexcitement, which can bring about a euphoria that seems initially to stimulate your sexual desire. With long-term, chronic use, however, the drug can ultimately cause you to lose interest in sex altogether or to become impotent.

Continued use of cocaine is damaging, and the symptoms of chronic cocaine abuse are serious. If you use cocaine, you can experience delusions of persecution, grandeur, jealousy or violence. You may also experience muscle spasms. If you use cocaine often, you will probably be constantly nervous, excitable, oversensitive to noise and susceptible to frequent mood swings, memory loss, compulsive scribbling (graphomania) and anxiety. You may suffer from auditory and visual hallucinations that make you think someone is persecuting or oppressing you. If you are a chronic user, you can be very dangerous to those around you, and may be capable of committing brutal crimes, or may even attempt suicide or homicide. In addition to mental disturbances, you may develop such physiological disorders as feebleness, emaciation, digestive disorders, nausea, vomiting, loss of appetite, a fast pulse or impotence.

Crack

Crack, as mentioned above, is created from pure cocaine during the freebasing process. Today, it is the drug of choice on the streets of America. Crack is processed in illegal laboratories in "crack houses" by mixing ordinary cocaine with a solution of baking soda or ammonia and

If you're looking to break your addiction to drugs, you'll be happy to know that you have many different options. Health experts and community service programs, such as Narcotics Anonymous (NA) and Cocaine Anonymous (CA) have developed three approaches to drug treatment—detoxification, maintenance and therapeutic communities.

- ◆ *Detoxification* means that you're taken off the drug as soon as possible. Your physical and psychological distress resulting from the withdrawal process is then treated.
- ◆ *Maintenance* usually means you are given a synthetic narcotic (methadone), which mimics the effects of the drug you have been using, but does not have the same side effects. The replacement synthetic drug allows you to wean yourself off the drug without the trauma of going "cold turkey," or stopping drug use immediately. This treatment is only effective only if you are addicted to a narcotic.
- ◆ Entering a *therapeutic community* is one way drug addicts have been able to successfully recover. In 1958, a former alcohol and drug addict, Chuck Dedrich, set up a new type of treatment center for drug addicts. He called it Synanon and modeled it on Alcoholics Anonymous, of which he had been a member. There are now more than 300 such centers throughout the country. Addicts at Synanon are called clients because they or someone else pays for the treatment, and all members enter the program voluntarily. Most clients are from a minority group; quite often they come from unstable homes and are poorly educated. The staff of Synanon is composed of ex-addicts, counselors and trained professionals.

heating it until the water evaporates. The residue from this "cooking" is crack, a solid crystalline substance that is then broken into pieces or chips. Two or three of these chips make a dose of crack, which is sold on the street for $5 to $25.

Crack is taken into your body by smoking the substance from a glass pipe. Many users also crush crack and smoke it like a marijuana joint. When heated, the chips crackle—thus the name "crack." Heating crack changes it to smoke, which is inhaled, drawn into your lungs and then diffused rapidly throughout your bloodstream. Your circulating blood transports the dissolved cocaine to your brain, where it takes effect immediately. Snorted cocaine reaches your brain in two or three minutes, but smoked cocaine reaches your brain in a matter of seconds.

The effect you feel when smoking crack is called a "rush," or a sudden high caused by the assault on your brain and central nervous system, which responds by stimulating certain body reactions: increased body temperature, involuntary movement of muscles, and overstimulation of the pleasure centers in your brain. Since the high from crack lasts for a short period of time, ranging from one to ten minutes, the drug is used up very quickly.

When the high level of chemical activity in the brain cells stops, a crack user will often experience a condition called a rebound. A rebound can happen with any form of cocaine. If you feel extremely depressed, lethargic or negative after crack use, there's a good chance you're experiencing a rebound.

Even after a short period of time, regular crack use will have abnormal effects on your brain. Your brain's pleasure centers will slow down. As your pleasure centers lose their ability to respond, you may decide to increase your dose of the drug in order to regain your rush or high. The attempt to get pleasure from the drug becomes so compelling that many addicts devote their entire lives to obtaining and smoking crack.

Effects of cocaine and crack

Here are some of the ways cocaine and crack can affect your body:

Blood vessels: Cocaine and crack can increase your blood pressure to such a degree that you can be at risk of having a stroke. In fact, doctors have reported an increasing number of fatal strokes among crack users.

Skin: Occasionally the skin on your face will get oily and become covered with pimples.

Eyes: As with heroin, cocaine and crack cause the pupils of your eyes to dilate and remain open. Your eyes then become sensitive to light, and your vision will become impaired during drug use. To reduce these problems, many crack addicts wear dark glasses constantly.

Heart: Using cocaine or crack will speed up your normal heart rate by 30 to 50 percent. Both drugs can also interfere with the regularity of your heartbeat, making it skip a beat and then do two rapid contractions to compensate.

Lungs: Cocaine and crack both inhibit the proper exchange of oxygen and carbon dioxide in your body and destroy your lung tissue and air sacs. Users of these drugs often develop bronchitis.

Muscles: Both drugs affect your muscles and cau tics or involuntary jerks. You may even suffer fr vulsions after using these drugs.

Treating drug abuse

If you're a drug user, your substance of choice, it's alcohol, crack or even nicotine, may very wel most important thing in your life. It's very like you don't want to quit. You probably get a lot of from the way the substance makes your body feel, for a while. After all, using drugs and alcohol can social. Your friends or family may not think you' "cool" if you tell them you want to stop. Howeve drug or alcohol use may also be ripping you apa those who care about you most, those who want be healthy and in control. Regardless of what h ation is, breaking an addiction of any sort could ve be the most difficult thing a man needs to do as a being. When it comes to your health and true hap seeking help is the strongest, most courageous thi can ever do for yourself.

John Lucas is one hero who overcame drug ad A former player for the Houston Rockets and covering drug addict, Lucas was given a second by the sports world when he was named coach San Antonio Spurs basketball team. In this new ca Lucas formed a counseling group to help other basl players and athletes like himself who had been b from participating in organized sports because o use. Today, Lucas uses many of the recovery stra he learned when fighting his addiction to guide h ketball team to victory.

Conclusion

The effects of substance abuse can be devastating—both to you, if you're an abuser, and to your friends, family and coworkers. If your life is so stressful or unpleasant that you must rely on a substance to cope, try to deal with the cause of the tension in another way. Sports, exercise or stress-reduction techniques can all help. Sometimes opening up to a family member, a close friend or even a therapist can help you find the support you need to make a change.

Abuse of any kind is hard to break, and finding the support you need is essential. If you are a substance abuser, remember you are not alone. Not only are there thousands of people in the same situation as you, there is also a network of confidential professionals who are willing to help. Take it day by day and set small goals for yourself. Seek assistance and reach out to your family and friends who care and are willing to offer guidance and support. You may be surprised how helpful others will be.

Your ultimate success will be up to you. You owe it to yourself to lead a long, healthy and happy life. Make a choice to give yourself the greatest gift you can ever give—health. Step by step, you can break your addiction. You just have to make the first move.

Resources

Al-Anon
One Park Avenue
New York, NY 10016
(800) 356-9996

(Al-Anon provides information and support for families of alcoholics, using the 12-step program.)

Alcoholics Anonymous
P.O. Box 459
Grand Central Station
New York, NY 10017
(212) 870-3400

(AA offers brochures, pamphlets and self help for those interested in recovery. You can find your local chapter in the white pages of your telephone book.)

American Cancer Society
777 Third Avenue
New York, NY 10017
(212) 586-8700
(800) 422-6237

(The Society offers free information, literature and referrals.)

American Health Foundation
320 East 42nd Street
New York, NY 10595
(212) 953-1900

(The Foundation offers self-help brochures.)

American Lung Association
1740 Broadway
New York, NY 10019-4374
(212) 315-8700

(The Association offers materials on smoking classes, as well as general pamphlets and brochures. Look up your local association office in your telephone book.)

National Clearinghouse for Alcohol and Drug
  Abuse Information
Box 2345
Rockville, MD 20850
(301) 468-2600
(800) 729-6686

(The Clearinghouse offers brochures and pamphlets free
to the public. Ask for their most recent catalogue of free
publications. You can also speak to a specialist about any
specific problems.)

Appendix

WORK-RELATED ILLNESSES

By Peter Davis

The following list is not intended to be complete but is intended to give the reader an idea of occupational hazards associated with each listed job. Ask your doctor if you have questions about symptoms that might match your occupation.

Bird handler: Ornithosis is a disease carried by birds that may be contracted by humans, resulting in a lung infection.

Blacksmith: Infrared light may cause vision problems.

Boot and shoe industry: People in this occupation may be at risk for cancer of the nasal cavity.

Bridge maintenance: The inhalation of spores or fungus may lead to lung infections like pneumonia.

Carpenter/cabinetmaker: Chemicals known as chlorophenols may lead to cancer of the nasal cavity. Hexane (another chemical) may cause inflammation of the nervous system.

Coal miner: Exposure to coal dust may lead to a disease called pneumoconiosis, which is a lung disease characterized by emphysema.

Coke iron worker: Coke oven emissions and tar distillates have been associated with cancers of the scrotum and kidney.

Coppersmith: Chemicals used in this industry have been associated with cancers of the lung and trachea.

Copper smelter: Inflammation of the brain, known as toxic encephalitis, may be caused by the use of lead. Symptoms include a stiff neck and mental confusion.

Cotton industry: Byssinosis is a lung disease caused by cotton, flax, hemp or synthetic dusts.

Cryolite workers: Workers may suffer from discoloration of teeth enamel due to excessive ingestion of fluoride.

Dry cleaners: A chemical called carbon tetrachloride may lead to toxic hepatitis, which is an inflammation of the liver. Symptoms include weakness and yellowing of the eyes or skin (jaundice).

Explosives industry: Certain chemicals used may cause diseases of red blood cells, resulting in fatigue.

Farmer/rancher: Many diseases may be encountered. Some important ones include: plague, transmitted by infected fleas; anthrax, transmitted through infected animals and causing open skin lesions; brucellosis, contracted from goats, cattle, pigs, and associated with headaches and malaise; leptospirosis, an infectious disease contracted from dogs, pigs, rodents or contaminated water that can cause inflammation of the brain.

Fire- and waterproofing: A chemical, ethylene dibromide, has been associated with inflammation of the liver.

Foam and latex manufacturing: Certain chemicals may cause allergies of the skin resulting in hives, or may cause asthma.

Forester/plant worker: Fungus in the soil may cause nodules in the lymph nodes or skin.

Foundry worker: Some chemicals have been associated with cancer of the lung, while others may cause inflammation of the brain.

Glassblower: Infrared light may cause vision problems.

Hunter/fur handler: As with the farmer, many diseases may be encountered, usually as a result of coming in contact with infected animals. Some diseases include: plague, usually acquired via infected rats and associated with high fever; tularemia, associated with skinning rabbits and causing high fevers; tetanus, in which a toxin causes the neck and jaw muscles to contract; and rabies.

Jewelry maker: Platinum or inorganic mercury may activate a person's asthma.

Leather industry: Copper sulfate may cause a destruction of red blood cells, resulting in fatigue.

Lumberjack: Repetitive body vibration on the job may contribute to "Raynard's phenomenon," or sudden attacks of cold and pain in the fingers or toes.

Medical personnel: Anyone working around sick patients should be aware of the potential exposure to diseases such as tuberculosis and measles, among others.

Metal workers: Chemicals such as mineral-cutting oils have been associated with cancer of the scrotum.

Mining: Silica and talc may be inhaled, which could cause a lung infection (termed silicosis) and result in breathing difficulties.

Nickel smelting: Nickel may be associated with cancer of the nasal cavity. Lead may be used, which can cause inflammation of the brain (and result in headache and mental confusion).

Paper industry: The inhalation of sulfur dioxide may lead to bronchitis.

Petroleum refiners: Soots and tars have been associated with cancer of the scrotum. Exposure to ammonia can cause bronchitis if inhaled in adequate amounts.

Pigment industry: Certain chemicals have been associated with cancer of the bladder and lung. Other chemicals, such as benzene and copper sulfate, may affect the number of blood cells, suppressing the immune system or causing fatigue.

Plant protection: Pesticides and herbicides have been associated with cancer of the lung and bronchus.

Plastics industry: A chemical, trimellitic anhydride, has been associated with asthma, bronchitis, and the destruction of red blood cells, causing fatigue.

Poultry processing: Cumulative trauma, for example repetitive cutting, may result in inflammation of the nerves in the arms.

Quarryman: Silicon may be inhaled, which could cause a lung infection (termed silicosis) and result in breathing difficulties.

Rayon manufacturer: A chemical, carbon disulfide, has been associated with inflammation of the nervous system.

Refrigeration industry: The inhalation of sulfur dioxide may lead to bronchitis.

Rubber industry: Certain chemicals (benzidine and naphthyltamine) have been associated with cancer of the lung and bladder. Workers in this industry may also be at increased risk for leukemia.

Sandblaster: Silica may be inhaled, which could cause a lung infection (termed silicosis) and result in breathing difficulty.

Steel industry: Workers may be at increased risk for lung cancer, but the cause is unknown.

Vinyl chloride industry: Vinyl chloride may contribute to "Raynard's phenomenon," or sudden attacks of cold or pain in the fingers or toes.

Weaver: Anthrax is a disease that may be rapidly fatal.

Welder: Magnesium used in this industry has been associated with cancer of the lung and Parkinson's disease.

Whitewashing industry: A chemical, copper sulfate, has been associated with red blood cell destruction, resulting in fatigue.

NOTES

Chapter 3

1. Shulman, Neil B.; Saunders, Elijah; and Hall, W. Dallas (1987), *High Blood Pressure,* New York, Macmillan Publishing Company, pp. 2–3.

2. Hall, W. Dallas; Saunders, Elijah; and Shulman, Neil B. (1985), *Hypertension in Blacks: Epidemiology, Pathophysiology and Treatment,* Year Book Medical Publishers, Inc., Chicago, pp. 106–112.

3. Greenberg, Joel, "Science/Medicine," *Los Angeles Times,* September 30, 1991, p. B3.

4. Klag, Michael (1991), "Association of Skin Color and Blood Pressure vs. Blacks with Low Socio-Economic Status," *JAMA,* vol. 265, pp. 599–602.

5. Shulman, Saunders, and Hall, *High Blood Pressure,* p. 45.

6. Ibid., pp. 14 and 15.

7. Ibid., pp. 85 and 86.

Chapter 4

1. *Healthy People 2000,* U.S. Department of Health and Human Services, February 21, 1991, pp. 392–95.
2. Ibid.
3. "Heart and Stroke Facts," American Heart Association, p. 23.

Chapter 5

1. *Healthy People 2000,* p. 442.
2. *Report of the Secretary's Task Force on Black and Minority Health,* U.S. Department of Health and Human Services, January 1986, p. 150.
3. *Healthy People 2000,* p. 458.

Chapter 6

1. Chinni, Madeline, "Menus for the Anticancer Diet," *Science Digest,* vol. 102, February 1994, p. 14.
2. *Healthy People 2000,* p. 418.
3. *Report of the Secretary's Task Force on Black and Minority Health,* p. 88.
4. *Cancer Facts and Figures—1993,* American Cancer Society, Inc., 1993, p. 21.
5. "Cancer's Seven Warning Signals," *Washington Post/ Health,* December 3, 1991, p. 25.
6. *Cancer Facts and Figures—1993,* pp. 10–18.

Chapter 7

1. "About Sickle-Cell Trait & Anemia," Sickle Cell Foundation of Georgia, Inc., p. 6.

Chapter 8

1. General Information on End Stage Renal Disease, USRDS, Annual Data Report 1990, p. 2.
2. The Magnitude of the ESRD Problem, USRDS, Annual Data Report, 1990, pp. 5 (chart) and 6.
3. Statistics on Hypertension, Diabetes and ESRD, National Kidney Foundation of Georgia, Inc., 1989.

4. Kidney Failure Statistics, National Kidney Foundation of Georgia, Inc., 1989.

5. Black ESRD Statistics, National Kidney Foundation of Georgia, Inc., 1989.

Chapter 9

1. "CDC, Employee Education, Business Responds to AIDS," *AIDS Prevention Guide,* "How to Use a Condom," pp. 7 and 8.

2. "CDC Hotline Information," as of January 1, 1993.

3. "CDC Business Responds to AIDS," *HIV/AIDS: Are You at Risk?* p. 7.

4. "Positively Aware—the Quarterly Journal of Test Positive Aware Network," *HIV A to Z,* Winter 1993, p. 4.

5. *Healthy People 2000,* section 19, p. 496.

6. Ibid., p. 498.

7. "Chlamydial Infections Study Group Implements Single Dose Regimen," *NEJM,* September 24, 1992.

8. "New Reports Make Recommendations, Risk for Resources to Stem TB Epidemic," *JAMA,* January 13, 1993, vol. 269, no. 2, pp. 187 and 188.

Chapter 10

1. Herd, Dennis, "Migration, Cultural Transformation and the Rise of Black Cirrhosis," paper presented at the Alcohol Epidemiology Section, International Council on Alcohol and Addictions, Padova, Italy, June 1983.

2. *Secretary's Task Force on Black and Minority Health, Black and Minority Health,* 8 vols. (Washington, D.C.: United States Department of Health and Human Services, 1985), 1:70–75.

3. Ibid., p. 136.

4. "The Third Triennial Report to Congress From the Secretary, Department of Health and Human Services, on Drug Abuse and Drug Abuse Research," 1991, pp. 2 and 3.

5. Ibid., pp. 33 and 34.

6. "The Twelve Steps and Traditions," Al-Anon Family Groups (1973), New York, p. 2.

7. Escobedo, Luis G.; Anda, Robert F.; Smith, Perry F.; Remington, Patrick L.; and Mast, Eric E. (1990), "Sociodemographic

Characteristics of Cigarette Smoking Initiation in the United States," *JAMA*, September 26, 1990, vol. 264, no. 12, 1550–54.

8. *Healthy People 2000*, p. 147.

9. *The Seventh Special Report to the U.S. Congress on Alcohol and Health, Secretary of Health and Human Services*, January 1990, pp. 33 and 34.

If you're committed to eradicating inequalities when it comes to blacks and good health, you are invited to become a member of

THE BLACK MAN'S HEALTH PROGRAM
An Arm of the International Society of Hypertension in Blacks (ISHIB)

ISHIB is a unique nonprofit organization dedicated to improving the health and life expectancy of ethnic populations in the United States and around the world. Founded in Atlanta, Georgia, in 1986 to respond to the problem of high blood pressure among blacks, ISHIB has since then broadened its mission to include the total spectrum of disease in various population groups. ISHIB has been involved in health screening projects in Africa, South America, and North America, and publishes a journal entitled *Ethnicity and Disease,* which publishes reports on diseases among different ethnic communities around the world.

Heart to Heart is an ISHIB program that brings children from underdeveloped countries to the United States for much needed heart surgery. Heart to Heart helps set up the entire project, from locating the child, to finding a hospital willing to offer free treatment, to finding a place for the child, the child's parent, and the child's own doctor to stay for the duration. The program treats children from all ethnic backgrounds. Also, the doctors that come from the developing countries learn new procedures they can apply in their homeland. Cultural exchange programs also take place. Currently, Heart to Heart has helped 22 children from other countries receive heart surgery.

Your $50 membership fee will go to support:
*Community Service*Research*Drugs for Low-Income Hypertensives*Quarterly Medical Journal*1000 Medical References*Monthly Newsletter*High Blood Pressure Brochure*Special Projects*Future International Efforts in Ethnic Health

----

Join Today! Keep informed
and committed to black health!

Membership dues are $50. Payment must accompany application and will cover dues for current calendar year (January 1 – December 31). Make check in U.S. dollars payable to ISHIB. Return form with payment(s) to:

ISHIB
2045 Manchester Street, N.E.
Atlanta, GA 30324
404-875-6263

Name _____

Address _____

City/State _____ Zip _____

Country_____Phone_____